Nursing: Study and Placement Learning Skills

Edited by Sue Hart

Series editor Karen Holland

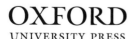

OXFORD
UNIVERSITY PRESS

OXFORD
UNIVERSITY PRESS

Great Clarendon Street, Oxford ox2 6DP

Oxford University Press is a department of the University of Oxford.
It furthers the University's objective of excellence in research, scholarship,
and education by publishing worldwide in

Oxford New York

Auckland Cape Town Dar es Salaam Hong Kong Karachi
Kuala Lumpur Madrid Melbourne Mexico City Nairobi
New Delhi Shanghai Taipei Toronto

With offices in

Argentina Austria Brazil Chile Czech Republic France Greece
Guatemala Hungary Italy Japan Poland Portugal Singapore
South Korea Switzerland Thailand Turkey Ukraine Vietnam

Oxford is a registered trade mark of Oxford University Press
in the UK and in certain other countries

Published in the United States
by Oxford University Press Inc., New York

© Oxford University Press 2010

British Library Cataloguing in Publication Data
Data available

Library of Congress Cataloging in Publication Data
Data available

Typeset by MPS Limited, A Macmillan Company
Printed in Great Britain
on acid-free paper by Ashford Colour Press Ltd, Gosport, Hampshire

ISBN 978-0-19-956312-8

1 3 5 7 9 10 8 6 4 2

Foreword

As newly registered nurses (mental health and adult) we both appreciate the enormity of starting a programme of nurse education, from the challenges we faced at university and in practice. In addition to the vast amounts of information to take on board in your first year, there are many books that promise to support you on your journey. We can both state wholeheartedly that we wish *this* book had been written when we were studying. But why do we say this and what makes this book different from others?

It contains all the essential information a student nurse needs to know in order to be successful in the first year, and presents this in a way that is accessible, lively and easy to read. It has been designed in such a way that the reader can dip in and out of specific areas that may be causing concern at a particular time. Alternatively, it can be read and digested chapter by chapter.

The student comments that have been used all the way through provide helpful ideas and insights that support the content of the book. Contributing student nurses who have recently 'lived' the experience shed light on the essence of being a student nurse, identifying what actually happens and how you can adapt to get the most from the course.

The advice given by the nurse mentors is imperative when starting placements as these can be daunting, especially if you have never worked in health care before. The explanations in the text about practice can hep alleviate stress for the new student nurse. This would have been an enormous help to us on our early placements and wish we could have read about these issues in this clear and simple way to support us before we began.

To reinforce your learning you can access the accompanying on line resource which gives another dimension to your studying; with interactive sessions to enhance your learning.

This book will undoubtedly help to guide, support and develop the flourishing nurse inside you. It will build your confidence through increasing your knowledge and understanding of the course and what you need to do to be successful. This book really does have the answers to all those unanswered questions that you have now as you start, and will have in the future. The first year of your nurse education programme is very challenging in many different ways and when you need help to support your learning this book will do just that.

Lastly we would like to say how proud we are to have been involved as 'student commentators' in the development of the book and that we are delighted to endorse it now.

Good luck on your programme.

Jo and Lisa

Jo Avery RNA, BSc (Hons), Staff Nurse, Surgical High Care Unit

Lisa Hawthorne RNMH Dip HE, Drug and Alcohol Service Community Nurse

(Pre registration Nursing Programme, September 2006 cohort University of Surrey)

For my niece Brittany Hart, a student nurse in Canada, and my father Brian Hart, for his unfailing support.

Series editor preface

Learning to be a nurse requires students to develop a set of skills and a knowledge base which will enable them to make the transition from learner to qualified nurse. As with any transition this can often seem at times to be a daunting prospect, and one where the student may ask 'how am I *ever* going to learn all that I need to know to get through this course and become a qualified nurse?'.

For student nurses this experience entails learning in 'two worlds', that of the university and that of the clinical environment. Although there is a physical distinction between the two, it is important that the learning that takes place in one is integrated with the learning in the other. This series of books has set out to do just that.

These 'two worlds' require that students learn two sets of skills in order to qualify as a nurse and be ready to take on further sets of skills in whatever nursing environment they are employed in. The skills which will be a core part of this series are numerous, and central to them is that of 'coping with the unknown'. For example, facing a new environment each time they start a new clinical placement, communicating with patients and a large number of health and social care professionals, dealing with difficult and often complex situations and sometimes stressful clinical experiences. In the university there are also situations which may be unknown, such as learning new study skills, working with others, searching and finding information, and managing workloads. It is every student's goal to complete their course with the required foundation for the future and it is the essential goal of this series to enable the student to develop skills for a successful learning and nursing experience.

The central ethos to all the books therefore is to facilitate and enhance the student learning experience and develop their skills, through engaging with a variety of reflective accounts, exercises and web-based resources. We hope that you as the reader and learner enjoy reading these books and that the guidance within them supports your goal of successfully completing your course of study.

Karen Holland

Series Editor

Preface and acknowledgements

If you have already begun, or are just about to begin, the first year of your pre-registration nursing diploma or degree programme, then this book is for you. In the pages that follow you will find information and guidance to help get you started. There is practical advice to support you through your first year of studying at university, as well as guidance to assist you through the practical nursing placements you will undertake during the first year 'common foundation programme'. The book has been written with the primary aim to help build your confidence and to support you to be successful. It does this by focusing on areas where we know students in the past have sometimes struggled and by offering practical advice and guidance. It is intended to be a book to carry with you into all your first-year placements, and into university, to dip into frequently and to re-read whenever necessary.

I am grateful to many people, students, colleagues, friends, family for their support and input at various stages during the development of the text. Thank you and apologies to anyone I may have unintentionally omitted.

Dru Rosenberg, Rebecca Lobb, Alicia Barrett, Jo Avery, Alison Sage, Mary Dearth, Cheryl Simner, Denise Mathews, Janet Nicholson, Keith Hart, Jenny Partridge, Jo Polley, Jemma Rhodes, Katy Gathercole, Kathy Curtis, Louise Heron, Rachel Williams, Rachel Griffiths, Nick Alexander, Faisa Nuur, Cath Moore, Lisa Hawthorne, Sam Brown, Sue Syer, Shelley Wilson, Zoe Creasy, Louise Salvi, Lisa Poynor, Dawn Carlton, Paula Battersby, Dimitra Theodosiou, Gala Dawson, Jane Pettingell, Nancy Hart, Glenys Tupper, Sarah Buringham, Simon Ralph, Shelley Wilson, Theresa Hughes, Donna Townsend, Lisa Greenwood, Alison Rose, Jackie Allen, Samantha Deveson, Lisa Millington, Hayley Scanlon, Sam Aitcheson and Debbie Croft.

Special thanks also to Emma Heaton (for the illustrations), Liz Rockingham, Debbie Roberts, Sheila Muller (for their chapters), Karen Holland (for sharing her experience so generously) and Geraldine Jeffers (for her patience and support). I am also grateful to the anonymous reviewers, current nursing students, mentors and nurse teachers from across the United Kingdom, who peer reviewed the manuscript and offered numerous helpful suggestions. It has been a privilege to work with you all.

Sue Hart
June 2009

Contents

→ GET THE ADVICE → DEVELOP THE SKILLS
→ PREPARE FOR PRACTICE

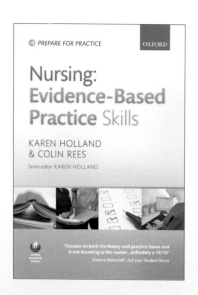
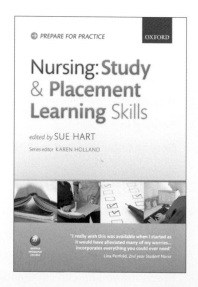

Nursing is more than just a job or simply studying at university and on today's nursing courses you need more than a standard textbook to support your studies.

With *Prepare for Practice* you'll find what you need to succeed. Get advice from those who have been there, find practical guidance for learning, assignments and exams, and find out how to maximise your placements to be truly ready for registration.

Visit the website for more tips, exercises, examples, and online activities
www.oxfordtextbooks.co.uk/orc/prepareforpractice

Smart nursing from Oxford

Detailed Contents

A word about the authors

Editor

Sue Hart is a mental health and learning disability nurse who has worked in nurse education for 18 years and, until 2008, was Director of Studies for the Common Foundation Programme at the University of Surrey. She is now a freelance educator. Sue has a particular interest in the health needs of people with learning disability, and has published numerous papers.

Contributors

Sheila Muller is a placement learning facilitator for Surrey NHS Primary Care Trust. She has worked in nurse education and research for over 20 years. Her teaching and research experience has focused on health promotion, smoking cessation, primary care, and the impact of a nurse education programme on the lives of mature students.

Debbie Roberts works at the University of Salford. She has been a lecturer in nursing since 2000, following 13 years in clinical practice. Debbie has published several papers regarding teaching and learning in nurse education and regularly presents at conferences. Her PhD research concerned peer learning: how and where student nurses learn from each other.

Liz Rockingham is a nurse tutor at the University of Surrey, where she is part of the Lifelong Learning Framework in the Centre for Research in Nursing and Midwifery Education. Her teaching includes study skills and mentorship.

Liz continues to work in clinical practice for part of her time, for the critical care service in a local NHS acute Trust.

How to use this book

Nursing: Study and Placement Learning Skills outlines the skills that first year student nurses need for success on their course. This brief tour of the book shows readers how to get the most out of this textbook and web package.

It's all new to me!

Find what you need fast! The detailed list of contents in the front of the book, and the chapter aims at the start of each chapter will help you find what you need, quickly.

What does that mean? You will come across lots of new technical and professional words in nursing. These are highlighted in blue in the text and explained in the glossary at the back of the book - you can also revise these online.

> erformance, with little modification or development. On the
> s a feature of the nursing profession, and to be successful, a
> ccommodate this fact.
>   The Nursing and Midwifery Council (NMC) (see Glossary)
> esponsibilities and duty of care nurses have to their patients
> he right to expect that the professionals nursing them are up-to

A word about This provides a more detailed explanation of a term used - for example explaining what exactly off-duty means!

> ••• **A word about** 'Off-duty'
>
> In the world of nursing, the term 'off-duty' refers to the r
> on-duty (the days and shift times you will be on the ward
> be off-duty (i.e. when your day/days off will be). The 'off-d
> nurse in charge. Off-duty might be done in advance for
> week at a time.

Practice and Practise

Throughout this book reference is made to the clinical practice area (with a 'c') and nursing practise (with an 's').

Practice is a noun, a person, a place or a thing.
"The student was looking forward to her first day in clinical practice." Here practice refers to the place where the student has been allocated.

Practise is a verb, an action word.
"The mentor made sure the student had the opportunity to practise the new skill." Here practise refers to the carrying out (doing) of the nursing skill.

Real world advice

Benefit from the experiences of current and former student nurses who give their advice on the course and placements!

Student comment

❝ Get a torch, as you will need one at some point, eve
tainly before you go on night duty. On a hospital ward,
the middle of the night using the light from your car key
patient wonders what you are doing crawling under thei

Succeed at university with tips from nurse teachers to help you to link university 'theory' and nursing practice.

Nurse teacher comment

❝ I am always upfront with students about reflectior
may find it hard, but that they all have the ability to do it
it comes naturally, others have to work at it. Once they
to reflect on things that go wrong or are difficult. I say

Succeed on your placements with key insights from registered nurses who teach and assess student nurses in placements (mentors).

Mentor comment

❝ If you struggle to identify learning goals of your ow
outcomes, then do not worry. Many placements will h
based learning activities that are open for first-year s

Helping you to develop your skills

Exercises Completing these activities will help your development, clarify an issue and get you thinking.

Exercise 6.2 Numeracy

Try the following eight questions (answers can be found at the
Key: X = multiply; / or ÷ = divide
1. 32 x 4 =
2. 1239 + 3178 =

Important facts at your fingertips Fact boxes provide essential helpful information and are easy to find.

! **Fact box** Examples of methods of assessmen
nursing programmes

Essays give you an opportunity to link experience in prac
been taught in class, literature searched and read about
onstrate your understanding by supporting your work with

Warnings Special boxes prompt readers to avoid common mistakes and to not forget key items.

 Avoid Making promises you cannot keep

If a patient tells you something that puts you under a stra
swallowing their medication when given it, and then asks
not promise this. Your duty is for the well-being of the clie
you may have that they may be cross with you for betraying
keep such a confidence is unfair to you; do not let it compr

Nursing practice examples It can be difficult to integrate theory and practice at first, so new nursing students will find these helpful.

Top tips Every chapter ends with practical suggestions and advice.

Online resource centre

Nursing students need to use a variety of online nursing materials throughout their course to find information and develop their skills—this book has a dedicated website to help you get started! Just save the url in your 'favourites' in your web browser and go there when instructed to in the book.

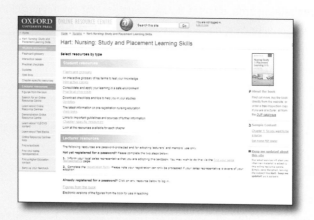

www.oxfordtextbooks.co.uk/orc/hart/

- Learn nursing terms quickly with the interactive glossary
- Download practical checklists for placement
- Save time by using the links to sources of further information and guidelines
- How will the review of pre-registration nursing education affect what students need to learn in first year? Find out using our updates
- For lecturers—you can download the figures for the book and use the resources in your classes

Introduction

How this book can help you succeed on your pre-registration nursing course

Whether you come to it straight from school, or as a career-change mature student, or after working in a health-related area, such as a care assistant, the pre-registration nursing programme can be very challenging, as well as exciting and stimulating. There is a great deal to learn, many new experiences to face, and numerous hurdles to cross.

It is *precisely because the course is challenging* that the idea for this book was developed. It has been written by three nurse teachers and a senior nurse. When developing the text, the writers collaborated with some recently qualified nurses, a group of current nursing students and a number of registered nurse mentors. We did this because we felt that there could not be a better placed group of individuals to advise and guide you through the first year of the programme, than nurse academics who teach the course, mentors who teach and support you in practice and a group of recent and current nursing students.

The book has been designed to be friendly and interactive and to 'speak' to *you* the student. Many textbooks you will need to read in the future, as part of your course, will be more 'academic' in their style. By this we mean supported throughout by many references to earlier works and to research. This book intentionally, is quite different in its approach.

Pause for a moment and imagine there was always close by you an experienced and wise nurse, excellent in practice, utterly professional and highly competent academically; a superb role model. You could turn to this person whenever you needed (day or night!) to help support you through the challenges, problems and conundrums you are faced with during your first year as a student nurse. What a comfortable thought, but how impossible in reality for such a situation to occur. Back in the *real world*, this book can be close to hand at all times and its goal is to help make your first year an enjoyable experience and builds your confidence.

A book for student nurses everywhere

This book has been written in England and for this reason certain sections (e.g. how health and social care are organized) have a United Kingdom focus. However, the majority of the text is intended to be as informative to overseas nursing students, as well as to those closer to home. Irrespective of location, the journey through the first year of a nursing programme encompasses the need to learn basic skills in clinical practice, to understand the theory on which nursing practice is built and to appreciate the importance of developing the necessary professional skills. The book has its primary focus on these key areas.

The structure of the book

The book has seventeen chapters organized into three parts.

Part 1 consists of Chapters 1 to 4 and sets the scene for new students of nursing, by explaining some of the basics about what the first day and the rest of the course will be like. It helps you to know who will be on hand to support you and how to find your way around. It contains a lot of helpful hints to help you settle and get yourself organized. It also introduces the three essential skills sets.

Part 2 consists of Chapters 5 to 15. These are all dedicated to helping you understand how to be successful in each skill area. Chapters 5 and 6 have their focus on the academic and learning skills you need to develop to be successful. Student nurses are adult learners and how you are required to engage in your learning is very different from school or college. Tips to enhance your study skills are included to enable you to get the most out of the course. In Chapter 7 the book starts your introduction to practice, by explaining where your placements will take place and introducing you to the NHS and other key areas of practice. Starting clinical placements can be a stressful time. Chapter 8 builds your confidence by explaining some of the many ways your nurse teachers will ensure you are well prepared with the basic skills necessary for practice.

Student nurses go into practice to learn. But how do you learn? Chapter 9 talks you through how you learn and how to get the most from your learning experiences. Mentors are important in your learning, but who are they, what do they do and how will you work with them? This chapter will explain. The days immediately before your first steps into practice can be nerve-racking. That is why we wrote Chapter 10. Read it before you go into practice to see what is coming and prepare yourself as well as you can. There is a lot you can do to ease your pre-placement anxiety and feel confident.

As you are reading this we know you have plans to enter a particular field of nursing, adult, child, learning disability or mental health. But what you will come to understand in time is that the boundaries between the fields of practice are often blurred and that registered nurses have a responsibility to all patients and clients. For this reason we have included in Chapter 11 an overview of all four areas. If you are challenged by nursing a person with mental health needs on an adult placement, your mentor may suggest you 'reflect' on this issue. But what does this mean? Chapter 12 explains this important concept in language you will understand.

You will have had experience of your written work being assessed before, but how is clinical nursing practice assessed? Chapter 13 explains how and offers a lot of advice about how to be successful. Your success on the programme is reliant on you developing the necessary professional skills and behaviour. But what does this mean and where do you start? Read Chapter 14 to understand what is expected of you as a student. Chapter 15 then unpicks the professional code for nurses to help your understanding of what will be expected of you once registered.

Part 3 is Chapters 16 and 17. As nurse teachers we know some of the areas students find difficult, and Chapter 16 addresses these head on and gives guidance to help you to problem solve in areas even beyond those discussed in detail here.

The last chapter is your springboard to the second year. Although it does outline what to do if you are struggling at this stage, it mainly prepares you for second-year studies. Why? Because if you have read the book so far and followed the advice, there is every reason to believe that you will be successful.

Please note that in the text 'he' and 'she' are used interchangeably to describe students, teachers or mentors. 'Programme' and 'course' are used to describe what you are studying at university or higher education institution (HEI). Although the NMC now refer to 'fields of practice' we have sometimes referred to the 'branch programme', as we anticipate that this term will be used in practice for some time to come. The terms nurse teacher, nurse tutor and nurse lecturer are also all in fairly common usage and these will be used interchangeably. To describe that part of the course where you are working directly with patients and clients the terms practice, clinical practice and placement will be used.

■ References

Nursing and Midwifery Council (2008) *The code: standards of conduct, performance and ethics for nurses and midwives.*

PART 1

Getting on!

So you want to be a nurse

Sue Hart

The aims of this chapter are:

➤ To explain why nursing is a continually changing profession

➤ To demonstrate why developing effective strategies for learning and studying are essential for your career as a nurse

➤ To introduce three essential nursing skills sets: academic and learning skills; clinical practice skills; and professional skills

If you want to be a registered nurse, you need to be aware of the characteristics of the profession and to understand what your nurse education programme will demand of you. To be successful, a student nurse must reach the required standard of performance with regard to their professional behaviour, clinical practice skills and in their academic studies.

Student comment

❝ New students need to understand that they don't have to make their mark or show their potential straight away. I remember when I started, I wanted to prove how much I wanted this and how keen I was to get stuck in. The fact was I didn't need to right away because the uni just wanted us to settle in first and meet people. Relax is all I can say, and everything comes so much easier! ❞

1.1 Nursing is dynamic

If it was possible to travel back in time to the 1920s, what you would see of a nurse at work then would bear little resemblance to the nursing practice seen today. Nursing has evolved from vocation to career, and now has its own evidence-base and professional standards. This means nursing has its own body of knowledge developed over time, and clear ideas, guidelines and standards about what constitutes good nursing practice.

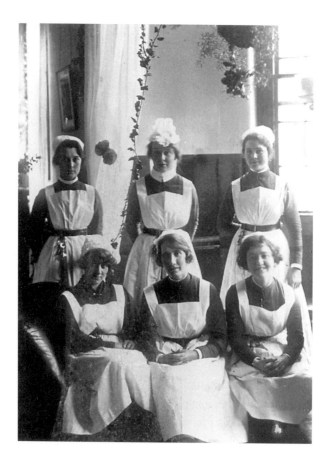

Figure 1.1 Nurses in the 1920s © Pie Powder Press

Developments in nursing are sometimes as a result of changes in the practice of another professional group. For example, a procedure once undertaken under general anaesthetic and requiring an overnight hospital stay for the patient, can now be performed as day surgery. This change has a 'knock-on' effect for nurses, as they need to understand the correct management of the patient following their treatment. To work with others, accept change and adapt is to grow into your practice. To resist change is to stagnate and, ultimately, to fail. If you seize the learning opportunities open to you now, you show your teachers that you are someone who looks as though they will 'fit' into the profession.

Why does nursing change all the time?

Imagine a conjuror performing a card trick. He fools the audience every time as the Queen of Hearts appears when they were certain, a moment ago, that he had put it back in the pack. Although quite difficult to learn, once mastered, such a skill can be rolled out at every performance, with little modification or development. On the contrary, constant change is a feature of the nursing profession, and to be successful, all registered nurses have to accommodate this fact.

The Nursing and Midwifery Council (NMC) code (2008) outlines the responsibilities and duty of care nurses have to their patients and clients. The public has the right to expect that the professionals nursing them are up-to-date with their practice, are competent and skilled to perform the tasks required, and are sufficiently knowledgeable to give the best possible advice and guidance.

To illustrate some of the ways nursing has evolved, consider the following from each of the four fields of nursing practice:

Adult:

- A conscious adult patient would have had their temperature taken with a mercury thermometer placed under their tongue.
- A patient's care plan would have been completed by hand and stored in a paper folder.

Child health:

- Sick children in hospital were separated from their parents, with only limited visiting times.
- Before special-care baby units (SCBU), many premature babies (i.e. born before the full term of 9 months) struggled to survive.

Learning disability:

- Known as mental sub-normality nursing, this took place in long-stay hospitals, the largest of which would accommodate up to 800 or more residents (Korman and Glennester 1990).
- The more able residents were known as 'high grades' and often acted as assistants to the less able 'low-grade' residents.

Mental health:

- Large psychiatric hospitals were the place most mental health nursing took place, and not in the community, as now (O'Carroll and Park 2007).
- Care was once mainly custodial with nurses meeting only the physical needs of patients and not their mental health needs.

(See Chapter 11 for much more about the four fields of nursing.)

In order to respond to the changing need for healthcare, many educational opportunities are offered, following registration. Most UK universities provide education for lifelong-learning, with opportunities to obtain higher degrees at masters and doctorate levels. Your pre-registration programme is just the start of an exciting career.

What changes ahead do we already know about?

At the time of writing, the NMC are reviewing the standards of proficiency for pre-registration nursing education and the first all-degree programmes are expected to be in place by September 2011. In the future there is to be a blend of generic and field-of-practice specific learning extending throughout the programme, with more field-specific learning increasing over time.

> **! Fact box**
>
> It is because nursing and nurse education changes so rapidly that this book has the online resource. If you are reading this *after* September 2011, you will find a link to the necessary updates you need, to support the information in the chapters that follow.

+ ·

Exercise 1.1

List 10 things that you think nurses of *today* do on a daily basis. Try to think beyond the obvious tasks (injections, bed pans, etc.). Also, do not just think about your own chosen field of practice. What do you think other nurses do? Refer back to your list when you have read Part 2 of the book.

· ·

1.2 Nursing: the life-long journey

Anyone planning to pursue a career that requires a minimum of 3 years full-time academic study and practice time *before* initial registration will have given a great deal of thought to the decision to apply for their course. When you were thinking of applying, you will have had your own thoughts about 'nursing' and what the course will be like, as well as your ideas of what it is that nurses 'do'. You may also have thought about the area of practice you would wish to work in once registered.

By now you will understand that over the next 3 years your goal is to learn, understand and develop the necessary nursing skills, and to acquire the essential knowledge needed to be successful in your programme of study and, in so doing, satisfy your teachers and mentors that you are a person 'fit' to be accepted on to the nursing register for your chosen branch.

What do you mean life-long journey?

In the past, once an individual was accepted onto the nursing register their nurse education effectively ended, with the exception perhaps of the occasional training course. Commonly, nurses referred to their 'ticket', meaning their eligibility to practise. Much as having bought a train ticket to travel from London to Manchester, the 'ticket' was the key to the job; nurses were not required to keep up-to-date with developments in their work, in the way they are now. Why would this matter? Patients would then not be getting the best, most 'up-to-date' care that they deserved.

The situation now is very different. The pre-registration programme is considered to be just the beginning of learning, and definitely not all you need to know. Also, when in clinical practice in the UK, student nurses now have 'supernumerary status' (see Fact box below) stressing they are there as learners, and not as a regular member of staff.

> **! Fact box**
>
> When as a student in your placement you are supernumerary, you are counted as additional to the established number of staff usually required for the area. This protects your time to be there to learn under the guidance of your mentor. Sometimes you will learn by observing and listening, at others by practising essential nursing skills. (See Chapter 9 for more information.)

The fact that registered nurses are required to keep up-to-date means that in the future, studying, reading journals and nursing text books, and going on courses will become an important part of your professional working life. You must have the evidence that you have done this in order to re-register every year with the Nursing and Midwifery Council. Failure to do so will mean that you will no longer be eligible to practise.

But I have only just started the first year!

Reading this as a new student you may feel we are leaping ahead somewhat, but we do so with good reason. It is helpful to know this now so you can, from the beginning of your course, recognize the value of developing efficient study skills and competence in your clinical work, not only to be successful in your pre-registration programme, but to be successful in your career.

From student nurse to registration and beyond

In the first year of the pre-registration programme, shared learning between students from across all the future fields of practice takes place. It gives grounding in the skills and knowledge essential for all areas of nursing. The later years of the programme are to ensure you learn how to deliver and manage the nursing care and skills in your chosen field: adult, child, learning disability or mental health.

Following registration as a nurse, there should always be opportunities to pursue further learning. This is known as continuing professional development (CPD) or life-long learning. An example of this would be courses at graduate or post-graduate level (e.g. a degree or a Masters in Advanced Practice). Depending on your field of nursing, you could further your study in accident and emergency or coronary care nursing practice, community learning disability nursing, neonatal intensive care or caring for people with enduring mental health problems.

1.3 **The characteristics of nursing**

Nursing is a diverse (varied) profession. There is no easy answer to the question, what do nurses do? The role and daily working life of a mental health nurse working with patients with Alzheimer's disease differs significantly from that of a paediatric intensive care nurse or community based diabetic specialist nurse. Learning disability nurses mainly work with people who are not ill. So, why are there such nurses?

Despite these obvious differences, it is possible to identify common characteristics across the nursing profession and it is helpful to understand these as you prepare for what is ahead.

Teamwork: nursing is one of several healthcare professions

Whatever the field of practice, most nurses do not work in isolation, they come into contact with patients, other nurses and professionals. For example, a learning disability nurse may need to liaise with a psychologist regarding a client's behaviour; a child health nurse may need to discuss a case with a paediatrician (a children's doctor). Working well with others, communicating clearly, liaising and valuing their expertise are essential to the effective delivery of patient and client care.

Where do nurses work?

If at random you asked a hundred people in the street 'Where do nurses work?', the chances are that a majority would say 'in hospitals'. Yet where nursing care is delivered has changed over time, and more and more patients are being cared for in their own homes, in specialist units, hospices, community health centres and walk-in clinics. Chapter 7 includes more information about where nursing care is delivered.

What does the patient/client want?

What the public expect from the National Health Service and the staff who work in it has developed over time. Health education, 'expert' patients (Department of Health 2001) and the concept of patient choice, all feature in the modern health service. People are encouraged to engage in their own care, and to discuss and agree this with nurses. Today nurses often speak of working in partnership with their patients and service users (and not just in mental health and learning disability nursing but all fields of practice). Nurses practice 'with' rather than 'do things to' patients.

1.4 So how do nurses do all this?

+··

Exercise 1.2

Pause a moment here and think about what you have just read. What do you think are some of the personal and professional qualities a nurse needs in order to perform their role effectively?

You may well have answered reliability, honesty, caring and good communication skills as some of the qualities, and there are many more. As you will have realized from the passages above, the willingness to face up to challenges, to communicate well, to liaise with colleagues and to be flexible are all important; but this is just the beginning.

Introducing the three essential skills sets

To be successful on the pre-registration nursing course it is fundamental that you understand the three essential skills sets, and appreciate why they are so important. It is because it is the evidence of your achievement in these areas which will, for the most part, indicate your suitability to become a registered nurse. Your success on the programme depends on you reaching a satisfactory level of proficiency in the following areas:

- academic and learning skills,
- clinical practice skills,
- professional skills.

Although listed above as three separate entities, in the 'real world' of nursing these skills overlap (see Figure 1.2). It is to assist your understanding as a pre-registration student in the first year of the programme that we present them separately here. Reading this book will help you to be successful in all three areas.

3. *Professional* standards required by the Nursing and Midwifery Council

1. *Theory* – that is the academic learning and understanding of the subjects which underpin nursing care

2. *Practice* – the undertaking of clinical nursing skills and nursing care with patients and clients

Figure 1.2 The three essential skills sets for nursing

The skills are equally important and you must achieve in all to be successful. The following introduces each individual skill set. Part 2 of this book explores them all in much more detail.

Academic and learning skills

As a university student and future registered nurse, you must be able to demonstrate through a variety of assessments that you have a basic understanding of the academic subjects underpinning nursing practice, such as biological science, psychology, sociology, nursing theory, ethics and care planning. It is vital that a registered nurse's actions are evidence-based. Also, as a student you will have to provide evidence (e.g. through reading nursing text books) to support your written work for the course. Chapters 5 and 6 will help you to develop the academic study and learning skills that you will need on the course. The second book in this series (Holland and Rees 2010) will help you to advance your skills in research and evidence-based practice.

Clinical practice skills

Clinical nursing practice (or 'practice') is the term that is used to describe the actual 'doing' of the nursing role. So whether you are supporting a patient to eat or drink, giving an injection, assessing someone who has a learning disability, working in an assertive outreach team in mental health, the 'doing' of these nursing skills is your practice. To be a registered nurse you must have the skills to perform your role. To be successful you must demonstrate through a variety of practice-based assessments, that you have the skills required to complete the first year and later the skills required for registration. Chapter 9 explains how you will learn in practice and Chapter 13 will help you to be successful in your practice assessments.

Professional skills

There are numerous differences between having a job and being a professional. Nursing is a profession. Once registered, you will be professionally accountable and responsible for your actions. The education and regulation of nurses, the existence of the nursing register, and 'The Code' (NMC 2008) are some of the strategies to ensure that only nurses who are fit to practice are able to do so. You will have a minimum of 3 years as a student nurse to show you can develop into the professional role. Chapters 14 and 15 explore nursing as a profession and outline what professional behaviour means.

Summary

Be confident. But also be aware the course can be challenging and this book is here to help. It tells you what you need to know to succeed. Settling in can take some time and Chapter 3 contains some healthy living and stress-busting mechanisms. It also gives advice about managing your money. The book will guide you through the essential skills sets to help build your understanding and give you the best possible grounding in the profession of nursing. Remember, if you can achieve the required standard in these three areas, you will be on the way to success. The first step to that success follows in Chapter 2, which is going to guide you through the first days of the course.

■ Top tips

- If you have been accepted on the course, celebrate—you have the potential to succeed.
- Settling in can take time.
- If you are worried or do not understand something ask.
- The nurse teachers are on your side and want you to succeed.
- Focus on developing in all the essential skills. Being excellent in practice but failing your exam is not going to lead to success.
- Writing excellent essays but never arriving in your placement on time is not going to lead to success.
- Enjoy learning, and not just for the assessments.
- Treat people in your care as you would wish to be treated.

■ Online resource centre

 To make the most of the advice in this chapter, and to develop your knowledge and skills further, now go online to **www.oxfordtextbooks.co.uk/orc/hart/** to find advice from other students and explore the Nursing and Midwifery website.

■ References

Department of Health (2001) *The expert patient: a new approach to chronic disease management in the 21st Century.* The Stationery Office, London.

Holland K and Rees C (2010) *Nursing: Evidence-based practice skills.* Oxford University Press, Oxford.

Korman N and Glennester H (1990) *Hospital closure.* Open University Press, Milton Keynes.

Nursing and Midwifery Council (2008) *The code.*

O'Caroll M and Park Q (2007) *Essential mental health nursing skills.* Elsevier Sciences, Edinburgh.

■ Further reading

The following are novels, each opens up the world of the people they are about.

Bayley J (1998) *Iris: a memoir of Iris Murdoch.* Duckworth, London.
   About a woman with Alzheimer's disease.

Faulks S (2006) *Human traces.* Vintage Books, London.
   A novel tracing the development of psychiatry.

Haddon M (2003) *The curious incident of the dog in the night-time.* David Fickling Books, Oxford.
   Written from the perspective of a 15-year-old boy with Asperger's Syndrome.

Picardie R (1998) *Before I say goodbye.* Penguin Books, London.
   About the mother of 1-year-old twins who develops cancer.

■ Websites

Department of Health: **www.doh.gov.uk/en/index.htm**

National Health Service: **www.nhs.uk**

Nursing and Midwifery Council: **www.nmc-uk.org**

Website about public services: **www.directgov.uk/en/index.htm?cids=Yahoo_PPC&cre=Store_Front**

Welcome to the course

Sue Hart

The aims of this chapter are:

➤ To suggest pre course activities

➤ To show the structure of pre-registration nursing programmes

➤ To guide you on your first day and during induction

If you have been offered a place or have already started the pre-registration nursing course, think of this as your first achievement. Not everyone who applies is accepted, and if you have been, this indicates you have the potential to be successful. Well done, and welcome.

This chapter will explain how the course is likely to be organized from the first day, through the induction to the end of the first year. It also outlines the role of some of the people you will be meeting. Based on the experiences of students who have gone before, the chapter introduces some of the challenges you may face and how to get support.

2.1 Before you start the course

We asked a nurse teacher how they would advise a student who has not yet started the course.

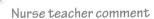

Nurse teacher comment

❝ If you have been offered a place you will most likely receive confirmation of this by letter and you must reply to secure your place. Study everything you are sent and respond to any instructions. You may be asked to fill in paperwork re a CRB clearance or be asked to attend an occupational health appointment. (If so, see 2.8 below for further information.) Reading through what you have been given will help you to find your way around your course and help you to understand aspects pertinent just to your own university/place of study. Also see the University website. If you want to live » *in university accommodation, apply now or you risk being disappointed. If eligible, you should also have been advised to apply for a bursary and, if you have not already done so, go to NHS Student Bursaries* **www.nhsstudentgrants.co.uk/** 🙰

Exercise 2.1

You have accepted your place on the course. Excellent! What can you do now to prepare yourself to start?

Read this book and others on a pre-course reading list. If your university offers a pre-start open day, do visit again. Ask questions. Some universities have online 'welcome' activities to bridge the gap between accepting your place on the course and actually starting. You will have been told if this is the case and have been given logon details.

••• **A word about** Pre-course reading

The nursing department may have given you a reading list. If the books are not in stock at your local library, it should be possible to order them. When you buy books take care to obtain those recommended by your nurse teachers and ensure you get the latest edition (your bookseller will advise). If you are instructed to buy a particular text book (e.g. anatomy and physiology) there will be a reason. It could be that exercises in class are based on the text. So you must buy them or else you will risk disadvantaging yourself.

Students come to pre-registration nursing from a variety of backgrounds. You may be joining the course straight from school or following a gap year, a former career or job you have been doing for some years. However, one thing is for certain; in the next 3 years your life is going to be very different from what it was before. Consider some of the ways:

- You will be studying and learning a lot of new things.
- You will be meeting many new people.
- You may have moved a distance from home.
- You may now be living some distance from friends and family.

Also, it is unlikely that before starting university you simultaneously needed to work on an essay, be on placement late in the evening and then up for an early shift the next day. How will your family manage this, let alone you? For new students time spent preparing for the change in circumstances will help.

Although it will have been explained during your interview day, it may help refresh your understanding of what you will be doing during your course to read the following overview of pre-registration nursing.

2.2 **Overview of pre-registration nurse education in the UK**

Wherever you are studying, your course has been designed to enable you to achieve the necessary proficiencies as laid down by the Nursing and Midwifery Council (NMC 2004) to become a registered nurse. The nurse teachers at your university, and their nursing colleagues in practice locally, will have written the curriculum (i.e. the programme of study) that you will follow. The curriculum will then have been scrutinized and approved (validated) by representatives from the NMC, your university and local NHS Trust. They must be sure that the content of the programme can help you to achieve the year one outcomes for entry to the branch programme and, at the end of 3 years, entry to the register (see the NMC website at **www.nmc-uk.org**).

Required hours for the programme

There is no 'national curriculum' for nurse education but, as the standards for pre-registration programmes are national, it follows that, wherever you are studying, there are certain essential NMC requirements to be met. Adult nurses must also meet the European Directives. The NMC stipulate that the pre-registration nursing course is not less than 3 years or 4600 hours in length. Allowing for any interruptions (such as ill health), full-time students must complete the course in not more than 5 years from initial registration and part-time students within 7 years. It is possible to 'step off' the programme and return later, as long as the maximum length of time is not exceeded.

The 3-year programme must be equally divided into 50% theory and 50% practice, and end with a 3-month period of clinical practice. It is usual that most of the 50% theory time takes place in the university, with some self-directed study. Normally the 50% practice time takes place in a variety of care settings in hospitals and the community. Up to 300 hours can take place in a university skills laboratory (see Chapter 8). In practice you will be required to experience 24-hour, 7-days a week opportunities.

At the time of writing, the NMC call the first year of the pre-registration nursing programme, the Common Foundation Programme (CFP). It is 12 months long and is the foundation on which the rest of the programme sits. It provides nursing students with learning opportunities in all four fields of practice (branches) and enables the acquisition and early development of essential nursing skills and knowledge.

See the online resource for this chapter where news of changes to the pre-registration programme will be explained after September 2011.

Entry to your chosen field of practice is by successful completion of the first-year outcomes required by your university, and by attaining the first-year NMC proficiencies (NMC 2004).

2.3 **How the pre-registration programme is structured**

Throughout the course you will be referred to as either being 'in theory', e.g. attending lectures, seminars or self-directing your own learning, or you will be 'in practice' being supervised by a mentor, experiencing nursing face-to-face with patients or clients, or undertaking other practice-based learning experiences, as agreed, such as a visit to a community learning disability or mental health service. When not in 'theory' or 'practice' you will be on annual leave, or possibly having a statutory day, such as a bank holiday. If you are sick, absent or on authorized leave, you will be doing so when you should either have been in theory, practice or on holiday.

> **!** **Fact box** Modules or units of learning
>
> Because what you need to learn to become a nurse is complex and varied, universities organize learning into discrete parts known as *modules* or *units*. These are independent units of study that combine to form your course. In year one you can expect to see titles such as 'Foundations of Nursing', or similar.

Figure 2.1 showing the theory/practice flow gives you an idea of how your first year may be structured. If you have it, refer now to the one for your course.

Your chosen field of nursing practice

We mentioned the four fields of nursing practice in the last chapter, and Chapter 11 says much more about them. On successful completion of the programme you will become a registered nurse (RN) followed by the field you studied, e.g. RN (Child). *The four fields are of equal status.*

> **⋯** **A word about** Changing from your original field of practice choice
>
> Most universities recruit students to join a particular field of practice and assume that students will not wish to change. In certain circumstances this may be possible, e.g. if you could do a direct swap with another student. If you wish to change, then tell your personal tutor as soon as you can. You may be asked to give good reasons so do your 'homework' before such a meeting is called.

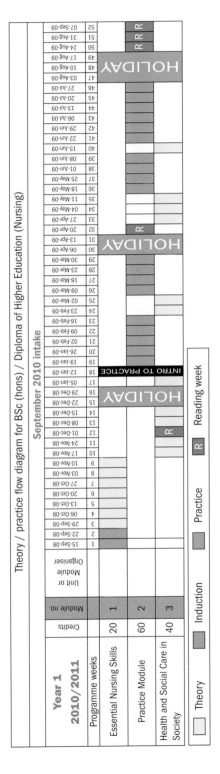

Figure 2.1 Example of a theory/practice flow diagram

2.4 **Students: how many on the course?**

How many students there are in your year group can depend on a variety of factors. For example, does the university have courses in all four fields of nursing at pre-registration? Some universities have one intake of student nurses every year, most often in September, others also have an additional mid-year intake in February or March. The autumn cohorts tend to be the largest.

If you are studying to be an adult nurse, invariably you will be a member of the largest group in your year. Adult tends to have the most students simply because more adult nurses are needed in the future workforce than nurses from the other fields of practice.

··· **A word about** The number of students on your course

> It is the future workforce planning needs of your local health care economy that determines the numbers of students being recruited for each branch. This is known as the sponsored (or commissioned) number.

2.5 **Starting the course**

We asked a number of current students what it felt like to start the course, what were some of the challenges they faced and how would they advise new nursing students to overcome them.

Student comment

66 I think one of the most important things to tell new students, is not to worry, as everyone else is in the same situation, and to try to be proactive in meeting people and chatting to people in lecture theatres, although this does come with time. I am still meeting people now who I haven't spoken to before. It's important just to be friendly and to be yourself, as you're all in it together! 99

66 For the first couple of weeks I would want new students to understand the message that, even though there is a lot take in, and settle in to, and the number of students you see everyday can be overwhelming, this is probably one of the very few chances to get to know the place, make friends (and make use of the student union bar!) because soon it is shiftwork and deadlines, and the chances may be more limited than they were at the beginning of the year. 99

The next part of this chapter is going to tell you something about what to expect on the first day of your pre-registration nursing course and outlines some of the likely induction programme activities. As the students indicated, to feel rather overwhelmed is not unusual; this would be an entirely normal reaction. Even if you feel that others look more confident than you feel, they may just be masking their own 'first-day nerves'. People manage in different ways. What is true is that you are all facing the 3 years ahead, and being supportive to one another to settle onto the course is important.

Nurse teacher comment

“ It may help you to know that the teachers in the nursing department at your new university are as pleased to see you arrive on your first day as you are to be there! They have invested a great deal already in getting you to this point and want to make you feel welcome and to support you to be successful. **”**

2.6 **Your first day at university**

Whatever the circumstances, when large numbers of people arrive at the same time at any venue it requires careful organization. On arrival you will find people around to welcome you and point you in the right direction. If you do not immediately see them, look for signs directing you or follow the map/instructions that you have been sent. Planning your arrival for at least half an hour (if not more) before the start time is good. This will allow for delays or getting lost. It also minimizes the chances (and embarrassment) of arriving late. All universities manage their new intakes differently but reading the following will give you a feel for what to expect.

Once you have arrived someone will advise you what happens next. Most likely this will be to be direct you to a lecture theatre big enough to seat students from all the nursing branches and possibly from other courses as well (e.g. midwifery, physiotherapy or social work). As all students need to be given the same basic information on the first day, and during the first week, it is practical to get everyone together for this purpose.

! **Fact box** Where to go on the first morning

At some point *before* your first day, the university will have sent information to tell you where to go on your first morning, where to park (if relevant) and how much it will cost. Do not forget to take this information with you when you leave home.

Nurse teacher comment

66 As CFP lead I organize the induction week and the welcome. My message always is to enjoy their first day. I stress the need to read everything we hand out. Many of the answers to questions new students have are in the programme handbook we give them. In a subtle way, I give the message right from day one, that they are adult learners, that this is a partnership. 99

Student comment

66 For me the big lecture theatres and the number of students were the scariest things, when I was in sixth form we only had about 15 students in each class. The way I got over that at first was by making a small group of friends and sticking with them when in big lecture theatres. 99

2.7 Induction (introductory) activities

It is common practice to start the pre-registration nursing programme with an induction and your first day at university is the first day of this. This will be designed to ensure you have all the necessary basic information required for your time on the course and to help you settle, explore the campus and locate key places, such as classrooms. Some universities run extended induction periods, from 2 weeks up to 1 month. These give your teachers time to cover basics, such as study skills (numeracy, literacy, note taking and essay writing)

• • •   **A word about** What to take with you on your first day

You are advised to take with you all the information you have been sent so far plus a few pens, a diary, note book and file paper. A note book is handy for jotting down room numbers and names of people you meet, and a diary for any appointments not on your timetable (e.g. to meet your personal tutor). File paper is good for any important information that you may need to refer to in the future, as it can easily be filed later. Different coloured pens can be helpful to differentiate sessions on your timetable. (See Chapter 4 for more about getting organized.)

to help prepare you for the course. They may also arrange a visit to the partner NHS Trust in which you will be doing your placements. A 1-week induction will just have time to cover the essentials you need to know, leaving topics (e.g. study skills) to be taught later.

> **!** **Fact box** Induction
>
> Expect to be sitting listening to people talking, for what may feel like long periods of time. If you are usually active, this can be surprisingly hard at first; but you must get used to it for the weeks ahead sitting in lectures.

The first welcome may be quite formal and from someone you may not see a lot of in the future, such as the head of the faculty. Later, talks will be from the people who are directly involved in your programme.

At some time during induction, expect to listen to presentations about fire, health and safety matters and security. If you are resident on campus or elsewhere in university accommodation, it is likely there will be advice particularly directed to you. The well-being of you and your fellow students is obviously a priority for the university and listening to the advice given makes sense.

Representatives from occupational health, the university counselling service, the library and IT support may also speak during the induction programme. Other talks may be from an NHS Trust representative, from 'professional bodies', such as the Royal College of Nursing (RCN) and possibly from the students' union. Just sit back and listen and later read any information handed out.

> **!** **Fact box** Paper
>
> It is stating the obvious to say that paper is expensive, photocopying in large numbers costly. It follows that if you are given paper copies, the university believes it justifies the expense. It suggests they want you to read, file it and refer back to it when necessary. At some point you will also be directed to access information through virtual learning environments (such as Blackboard, Web CT, Moodle and so on; see Chapter 5).

2.8 Other likely induction-period activities

Registering with the university

This may be done online or involve filling in paper forms. This activity is important as it puts you on to the central university database, gives you your student number and makes you 'officially' a student of the university. You cannot start the course, logon to the computers and get your university email address, and access the library, get your campus card or other ID, parking permit and so on, until you have done it. Expect to be asked for the name of someone who can be contacted in case of an emergency. Make sure you have the person's agreement, telephone number and address to hand. *It is essential that you do not miss registration.* If you have to for any reason, you must let a member of staff know so that alternative arrangements can be made.

Criminal Record Bureau (CRB) check

Note that this may happen during induction for some, for others before starting the course. Universities vary in their procedures.

All student nurses must declare any criminal conviction and, prior to interview, you will have agreed to a police check. Before you can start in practice you must be cleared by the CRB. You must provide evidence to confirm that you are who you say you are, and you will need, for example, to show a birth certificate or passport and to give details of your previous addresses. Your university will advise about this and how to complete the form.

Do not worry and assume that if you had a minor conviction some years ago this will prevent you from continuing on the programme. This is not necessarily the case. There will be a 'CRB counter signatory' or similar role title who will be able to advise you. The report back from the CRB is confidential. If you have had a minor conviction in the past, this should not become common knowledge to all your teachers, but only to the CRB counter signatory. If the CRB reveals a student with a record of certain serious convictions, they may be asked to leave the course or, if the CRB check was done in advance, they will not have been permitted to start.

Occupational health clearance

You are considered fit to go into practice following consultation with an occupational health department/health centre for screening. Like the CRB checks, this may happen either before you start your programme or soon afterwards. Failure to attend could mean a delay in going out to placements and later problems if you then run out of time to complete your placement hours. You could try to change your appointment if it clashes with a lecture or other session, but if you cannot do so, you must attend when asked. Occupational health nurses are there to support and help you, not to judge you.

!　Fact box　How to recognize which group or cohort you are in

For organizational purposes all groups must have a name, and it is customary to use the month and year the course started for this, e.g. 'September 2010'. A further means of splitting up the group is by future branch choice (e.g. child nursing) and programme followed, e.g. 'Jimmy Singh' Child Branch Degree, September 2010.

Uniforms

All universities manage the obtaining of uniforms differently. You will be advised. (See Chapter 10 for more information about uniform and Chapter 14 about appearance.)

2.9 Brief overview of subjects covered during the CFP

Wherever you are studying, certain key areas will be taught in the CFP. Nurses must have an understanding of anatomy, physiology and biological science, and psychology and sociology, as applied to nursing and healthcare. You will need to understand theories of communication and how health and social services are organized, as well as the roles of professionals who make up the multi-disciplinary/multi-agency teams (see Chapter 8). Health promotion is another important area. Planning the care of your patients and clients will be taught, as well as the skills necessary to practice within professional codes and guidelines. Ethics, law and social policy are all subjects likely to be taught in the first year. Chapter 9 says more about the teaching and learning methods used in practice.

2.10 Other useful information

Students with a disability or special need

Most universities operate a philosophy of 'self-definition' of any disabilities and special needs of its students. In other words, it is your responsibility to draw to their attention any particular needs you may have in order that the correct support systems can be put in place. The Disability Discrimination Act (2005), exists to protect people with disabilities and health conditions from unfair discrimination. The university has a duty in law to ensure its procedures are fair and to ensure that all disabled students can access all the areas that other students can.

For a pre-registration nursing student, the issue is whether once registered you would be capable of safe and effective practice, and it will be for your university and the commissioning NHS Trusts to consider individual circumstances. See the Disability Rights Commission website **http://www.drc.org.uk/** for further information.

Students with dyslexia

If you know that you have dyslexia or other difficulties in learning, make this known to some-one. Your programme handbook will explain what you need to do. Otherwise search your university website or ask to speak to the special needs representative in your department. You must make your needs known in order to qualify for special examination arrangements or the Disabled Students Allowance (DSA) in order to receive any equipment for which you may eligible.

Mature students with dyslexia

Some very able students come to university having managed through school with their diffi-culties with writing without having been assessed for dyslexia. If it is suggested that you are assessed, it is in your best interests to do so in order that the necessary support systems can be put in place.

Evaluations of taught sessions

Nurse teachers always work to improve their programme and receiving feedback from the 'customers' is important. Sometimes evaluations are done in groups, with notes made as you respond to questions about what you have been doing. At other times you will be asked to complete an evaluation form. If you want your comments to be considered, it is impor-tant to fill these in carefully following the instructions given.

Student representation and participation on the course

Your group will be asked to nominate one or more student representatives. Most courses have staff/student meetings, where students talk about any difficulties or make other com-ments they have about the course. Student representatives also attend more formal meet-ings such as boards of study. These are rewarding roles, as you help shape how your course is developed and learn more about your programme from the teachers' perspective. It also looks good on your future curriculum vitae (CV) as well!

Summary

This chapter has explained a lot of what you need to know to make a good start and to feel confident at the beginning of your programme. The next chapter is going to give you some advice about settling in.

■ Top tips

- At a minimum it is a 3-year course you are on. Take time to settle in.
- The first days can be nerve-racking: do not let it put you off your chosen career.
- Keep calm; deep, steady breathing helps.
- Remember, you are all newcomers in the same boat.
- Read all the paper work you are given and see Chapter 4 for helpful hints about organizing yourself
- If, having done this (and looked at the department website), you still do not know the answer to your query—ask for help.
- The course is not a competition, everyone can do well.
- Make friends and support each other.

■ Online resource centre

 To make the most of the advice in this chapter and develop your knowledge and skills further, now go online to **www.oxfordtextbooks.co.uk/orc/hart/** to read important updates on nursing education and to explore useful websites, such as the Nursing and Midwifery Council, the Royal of College of Nursing and more.

■ References

Disability Discrimination Act (2005) The Stationery Office, Norwich.

NMC (2004) *Standards of proficiency for pre-registration nursing education*. Nursing and Midwifery Council, London.

■ Further reading

Your programme handbook (read through electronically if you do not have hard copy).

Start reading texts from your first unit reading list—they may include books such as:

Garrett L, Clarke A and Shihab P (2007) *Get ready for a&p for nursing & healthcare*. Pearson Education, UK.

Hinchliff S, Norman S and Schober J (eds) (2008) *Nursing pratice and healthcare: a foundation text*, 3rd edn. Hodder Arnold: London.

■ Websites

Equality and Human Rights Commission: **http://www.direct.gov.uk/en/DisabledPeople/ RightsAndObligations/DisabilityRights/DG_4001070**

NHS Student Bursaries Home Page: **www.nhsstudentgrants.co.uk/**

NMC website at: **www.nmc-uk.org**

Settling in

Sue Hart

The aims of this chapter are:

➤ To provide tips for healthy living and healthy finances

➤ To understand how you will be supported

➤ To understand why good communication is very important

➤ To consider what you bring to the course

This chapter starts with a focus on you. If you want to care for other people, you must think about your own health, so that you are fit and well enough to do this. This chapter also explores how your attitude to the course and your behaviour can impact on your success (or otherwise). It stresses why communication with your teachers and mentors, who are there to support you, is so important. Whether you have just left home to start this course or you are a mature student with lots of life experiences to draw on, some of the following may help. Take from it what you need.

3.1 **Healthy you**

The message is simple: if you are going to look after other people you need to look after yourself. Taking care of yourself will improve your chance of success on the course. What follows are some healthy living *suggestions. If you feel you would benefit from reading these please continue*. If not, go straight to 3.2.

Eating

Breakfast is a must, plus at least two more meals a day. If you are working on a busy unit or out in the community, looking after other people, you will need energy (which comes from your calorie intake). Aiming to eat five portions of fruit or vegetables every day is good. If you enjoy it, then eat fast food/junk food as a treat, not a lifestyle. Good for you, and inexpensive, are jacket potatoes, raw carrots, watercress, apples, bananas, eggs, whole meal bread, yoghurt, nuts and tinned fish.

Watch your weight

Both being too slim or too heavy can be problematic. If you are failing to give yourself the necessary nutrients, you may lack the energy to perform well in practice and to concentrate in class. Conversely, if you carry a lot of extra weight, your body has to work harder to be active and you may be too weary to complete all your tasks. Occupational health will advise. See more information at the online resource.

Drinking

Try to drink at least six glasses of water a day. (If you do not like water, then dilute fresh fruit juice with water as a second-best option.) Enjoy alcohol, caffeine and sugar-rich carbonated drinks *in moderation only*. Some non-alcohol days are good for your liver. Restricting your use of caffeine as a stimulant is wise; use herb/fruit teas and decaffeinated coffee as alternatives.

Smoking

You do not need this book to tell you it is best not to; just read the packet. If you must do it, then do so in moderation only, and plan to stop. Seeing **www.nhs.uk/gosmokefree** will be helpful.

> **? Stop and think**
>
> If you are on a hospital ward and you smoke during your break in practice, then you must use a breath freshener and wash your hands thoroughly to remove any smell before going near patients. If they are unwell, the smell of smoke from you could be difficult for them to cope with and may cause nausea.

Illegal drugs

The use of illegal drugs of any type can be dangerous for your health and, if discovered, put your future as a registered nurse in jeopardy.

Rest

Getting enough sleep and quiet time is essential. Before lectures, or going into clinical practice, aim to get as many hours sleep as you know is good for you. However busy you are, try to have at least 10 minutes every day doing nothing. Just stop, relax, recharge your batteries.

Stress

This is better dealt with using healthy, rather than unhealthy, techniques. Stress happens for a reason; getting help to work out why you are stressed is the best way to approach it. Avoidance, increased alcohol consumption or smoking to try to combat stress are not helpful, and may make matters worse (Davis *et al.* 2008).

Nurse teacher comment

66 If you are upset by an incident in practice, talk to your mentor. It may also help to talk it through with friends (remembering confidentiality). If you are still worried, then talk to your personal (or liaison) tutor. See more about these roles below, and in Chapter 9. If your difficulty is of a personal nature, then see a counsellor. Most universities offer free or reduced rate counselling services for students. Remember, it is not just having the problem but how you *deal with the problem* that is the issue. 99

Exercise

Exercise is good for your body and mind. If you are physically tired after a day in practice, a short walk in the fresh air, swimming, cycling or yoga would be good. Try to develop good habits and keep them.

Have fun

You are on a tough course, which at times will stretch you physically, intellectually and emotionally. Plan your time out as you plan your work (see Chapter 4). See a movie, spend time with friends and talk about things other than the course. Give yourself a break, and be surprised how much better you feel afterwards.

As a registered nurse you have a professional responsibility to deliver care based on the best available evidence (NMC 2008). You will be more credible when giving health-promotion messages to patients and clients if you look like you care for yourself.

> **! Fact box** Sick leave
>
> If you are unwell, you must take the time you need to recover. It is your responsibility to do so. But do note that your sick days on the course are recorded and will be asked for by a future employer as a matter of course. If you *abuse* sick days and take them here, there and everywhere, this is not going to give a good impression. In the worst case scenario the employer may give the staff nurse job to someone else with a better record. Nurses have got to be reliable. You may look like you are not!

3.2 **Healthy finances**

Student comment

❝ When the loan comes through at the beginning of term it's easy to feel like you have a lot of money. Try to resist the temptation to spend it all, as you will find you really need it in the last few weeks of every term! ❞

Many students struggle with their finances when on the pre-registration programme. Difficulties can result from taking a drop in income, a lack of experience in budgeting or, for some, from sending money overseas to support their family. A National Union of Students (NUS 2008) survey found that students underestimate the costs of university life by up to £500 per year, and that the majority have to do additional paid work.

Important note

Be alert that too much extra paid work can detract from your studies: *do not do so much that you risk failing the course.*

Student comment

❝ When out shopping I have a think about whether I *want* it or need it, and if the answer is *want*, then I don't buy it. It gets quite boring after a while but does the job. You can cut corners by taking a packed lunch everywhere you go. ❞

»

66 I have a mortgage and two small children. The big thing is the child care, which you can claim for on the diploma programme. Although means-tested it helps massively and is in fact the difference between being able to do the course or not. It's important to budget and live within it. Make sure you get all the discounts, such as the council tax. Parking is a big issue with me. It was £160 per year at uni and then another £50 at hospital and then out in the community I had to pay to park in car parks. This takes a big wedge out of your money, so it's worth looking for places to park before practice. Car-sharing is a good way to save on petrol and sometimes the car park. 99

66 Doing some bank shifts for a hospital and a nursing home as a healthcare assistant has helped me. You can apply for a student loan, which is paid back once you are working again. If you Google student loan or go to your local council there is plenty of advice to be had. A bit of advice though is to make sure you do not encroach on uni time and work… it's better to go without rather than not complete work or, worse still, fail something. 99

What help is available?

Many nursing students are eligible for an NHS bursary. Contact the NHS Grants Unit (**www.nhsstudentgrants.co.uk/**) for information. You do not have to repay a bursary. If you are an older student with dependants, make sure that you are getting all the available allowances for which you are eligible from the NHS Grants Unit (such as tax credits or child care). Note the rules are different in the four countries, so you will need to check this.

Otherwise a student loan is one of the cheapest ways to support you through university. At the time of writing, these only have to be repaid once you are earning £15,000 at 3.8% interest. The current maximum is £4625, increasing to £6475 for London-based students. Anyone on an eligible course can get 75% of the maximum loan, the remainder being means-tested. It is possible to apply for a top-up from your local authority or the Student Loan Company (**www.slc.co.uk**).

Dependent on your household income and personal circumstances, it may be possible to get a maintenance grant (currently worth between £50 and £2835). Special support grants of up to £2835 are also available to fund child care, travel and equipment for the course. If you have a spouse or children, the child care grant, adult dependants' grant, the parents' learning allowance and the lone parents' grant are all means-tested grants available through the Student Loans Company or your local authority. You can also claim back essential travel costs, such as getting to placements (beyond £290). The disabled students allowance exists to cover additional costs you may have.

Most universities will have a hardship fund to which students with serious financial difficulties could apply for a loan. Some offer bursaries for students struggling financially, see 'bursary map' at the **direct.gov.uk** website.

Nurse teacher comment

66 If you are receiving an NHS bursary, you will be eligible to claim travel costs to and from your placements over certain miles (normally miles exceeding your home-to-uni-distance), either using your car or public transport. 99

See the money doctors!

This term refers to a training course sponsored by the Financial Services Authority to support university students to become 'financially capable'. Several universities have money doctors' courses. Your student services office or student union will advise.

+..

Exercise 3.1

Find out if 'money doctors' are running courses at your university. If so, the best time to attend is early on, in the first year. Then you have more time, and also it helps to learn about good money management sooner rather than later.

....

Other money tips

Surfing the net looking for ways to save money will repay in saving the time you spend doing it. Price-comparison websites are helpful for getting good deals for your mobile 'phone, computer, etc. (e.g. Gocompare.com, Uswitch or Compare and Buy at **www.guardian.co.uk**). Supermarket price-comparison sites (e.g. Mysupermarket.com) can guide you to the cheapest outlet for your basic foodstuffs. Money-saving expert websites (**www.moneysavingexpert.com**) also can be helpful. Always explore whether what you need is available through an online auction (such as eBay), rather than buying it new. Pick up discount vouchers when you see them and use the '20p off your next purchase' type offers. Even if you do not need them at the moment, buy non-perishable products when they are in a 2-for-the-price-of-1 offer. Look at **Raileasy.co.uk** or **Megabus.com** for good public transport deals. **Freebiesbank.co.uk** has free goods!

There is a lot you can do for yourself to settle on to the programme, but you will need the help and guidance of many people if you are going to be successful. What follows, explains who's who and how this will happen.

 Links to these can be found at the online resource.

3.3 **Who will support me to succeed?**

Some of the following you will get to know well, such as teachers and mentors. With others, such as support staff, placement officers and so on, your dealings will be mainly via email and telephone. The following explains the roles of people who will support you through the course. Be aware that some of the following role titles may be slightly different where you are.

University-based support

Programme lead

Whatever their title, it is usual for one person to be responsible for the *entire* pre-registration programme. Find out the name of this person in case you need to contact them in the future.

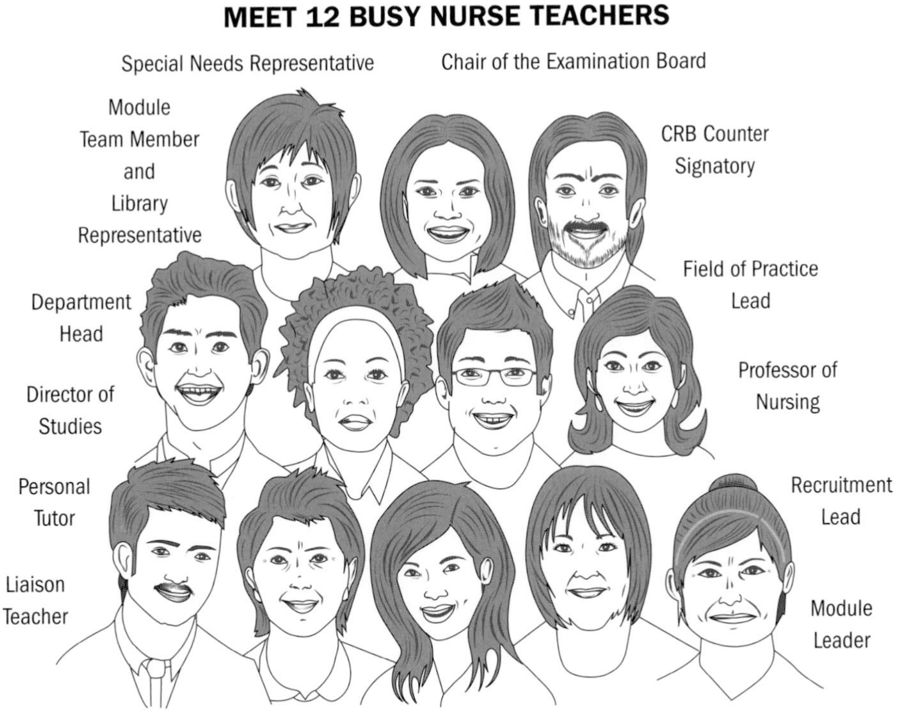

MEET 12 BUSY NURSE TEACHERS

Figure 3.1 Nurse teachers' additional roles. Artist: Emma Heaton

University-based nurse teachers

Teachers have various job titles (tutor, lecturer, senior lecturer, principal or clinical lecturer). Ask at your university about the differences, as there is no standard definition. Nurse teachers will all be on the nursing register, will usually have higher education qualifications (such as a Masters degree) and normally will have done a course to qualify them to be a teacher. Some may have studied for a PhD (doctor of philosophy). Professors are experts in their own field and, along with senior nurse practitioners, lead the development of nursing. You may be taught some subjects by non-nurse teachers, such as sociologists, psychologists or biological scientists.

In many ways the term 'nurse teacher' does not do justice to the variety of the role these individuals perform. Many are involved in practice development, research and writing articles for journals and books. See below and Figure 3.1 to understand why they always seem so busy.

Personal tutor

It is usual for all students to have a named personal tutor (PT) who supports and advises a group of personal tutees. In some universities, a PT may offer support with regard to personal, as well as course-related, difficulties, if these are affecting your studies. Your PT will direct you to sources of advice. Personal tutors generally like to see their tutees by prior arrangement for an occasional one-to-one meeting, and at other times in a group. It is very important to have the contact details of your PT easily available; you never know when you may need to contact them. *You must contact your PT if you are having problems.*

+··

Exercise 3.2

Find out all the important telephone numbers you will need to know: your personal tutor, the number to ring if you need to report sick, the library to renew books and put these in your 'phone or in a notebook. Today!
   Do the same with email addresses on your computer.

··

Module or unit leaders

The programme will be organized into blocks of learning called modules or units. Module or unit leaders have personal responsibility for planning the content, organizing the timetable, devising the assessments, and marking and moderating written work. Also, they will liaise with external examiners and the examination office staff. Once the teaching is completed, they will evaluate the module and, based on the feedback, recommend developments to the module, to the programme management team, board of study or other group who oversee the course.

Module or unit teams

These teachers work with module leaders to deliver the module. All teachers will be members of one or more module or unit teams.

Field-of-practice leaders

This teacher must ensure that the branch for which they are responsible is represented in the first year, as well as in the second year and beyond. They must ensure there are sufficient learning opportunities to enable all the outcomes for year one to be met.

Link or liaison teachers (both terms used)

Most nurse teachers are also link tutors to designated clinical placement areas. Wherever you go in practice there should be a named 'link tutor'. Part of their role is to support students in situations where they may be experiencing difficulties.

Special needs representatives

This person ensures that students with disabilities and dyslexia or other additional learning needs are directed to get the extra support they need.

Lecturer practitioners

Some universities and NHS Trusts jointly appoint nurses to work some proportion of their time (often half) in practice and the remainder in nurse education. For example, a registered mental health nurse may work 2.5 days per week as a community psychiatric nurse (CPN) and 2.5 days as a mental health nurse teacher. If your personal tutor has such a post, you will need to know the hours they work.

University-based support staff

Nursing programmes could not be delivered without these people, who perform a range of duties. They prepare programme and module handbooks and ensure that they are available (hard copy or electronically, whichever system your uni is using). Other support staff will keep the department website up-to-date and prepare the timetables. You may have already been given a uniform and a badge and it is likely that members of the support staff were involved in organizing this to happen.

Placement departments

These people may be called 'placement officers' or something similar. In collaboration with nurse teachers they determine where you need to go in practice, make contact with the placement and prepare the list of allocations. These lists are sometimes referred to as 'change lists'.

Exams office staff

Yet another team of support staff run the examination office and, with the teachers, over-see all aspects of your programme assessments, the schedule of submission dates and organize the exam boards and ensure you get the result of your work on time.

Clinical practice-based support

Mentors

Mentors are often, but not always, nurses (see Chapter 7) who have undertaken a mentor preparation course; they will guide, support, teach and assess you in your placements. As a student nurse, whenever you are out in a placement your named mentor is accountable for everything you do, although this does not stop the need for you to be personally account-able and responsible for your actions. See more about mentors in Chapters 9 and 13.

✚ ....

Exercise 3.3

You may also meet other staff with titles such as 'practice placement managers' or 'practice placement facilitators'. Find out what they do and how they can help you.

....

3.4 **How to find out what you need to know**

You will not succeed on the programme, and be where you need to be, unless you under-stand what information is essential and *where to locate* it. All universities manage information-sharing differently. Most now have a student website, which will have pages for your group, your timetable, copies of lecture notes for pre-reading and so on. Sometimes essential information may be handed out in hard copy in lectures. For instance, you will *probably* be given a paper copy of a programme handbook early in the course and reading this will be a source of valuable information and advice.

Notice boards or plasma screens are used to display important information (e.g your class timetable) and alert you to any unexpected changes on the day, such as a cancelled lecture. It is a good habit always to check these on the days you are in the university.

Later in the course you will need to find out where you are going to for your placements, also where to look for the results of your examinations and assignments. Your teachers will explain where you can find this information (possibly on notice boards and/or the student website).

3.5 **Communicate, communicate!**

Keeping in touch with the university: some guidelines

Sometimes the uni may need to write to you at home with important information. It is *essential* that you notify the department of any change in your home address. *In the long run failure to do so may disadvantage you.*

Other information may come to you personally, or to the entire group by email. So make it your habit to check your university email inbox whenever you logon. Also, look at the student website for any 'news'.

If your university is using a virtual learning environment (such as Blackboard), also get used to logging-on there regularly.

There may be 'pigeon holes' where alphabetically by surname you can pick up correspondence addressed to you. If you are given one, check your pigeon hole regularly.

There will be times when you will need to contact the university, e.g. if you are unwell and need to miss a lecture. You may have to miss lectures for other reasons, such as a family illness or bereavement. How you need to manage these situations varies according to the circumstances. The following may be helpful:

- If you are unwell on the day of an examination *speak to someone in person before the start time of the exam.* If you are very unwell, ask someone to telephone on your behalf. If you do, and later provide a medical certificate, there is a chance that your non-attendance will be discounted (which is to your advantage). Failure to communicate your absence in good time may mean you are awarded zero. This means you would have to sit the examination as if you were doing it as a second attempt (you lose your first attempt).

- If you are unwell on a Monday, and know you will be away for a week at least, and are due to see your personal tutor on Friday, an email to explain the situation and apologize for not attending would be acceptable. You are allowing enough time to expect your PT to have read the email.

- If you are ill on a Monday morning and had been due to see your PT that afternoon, a telephone message (to their voicemail or via a member of the support staff) would be better.

We asked a nurse teacher to talk to us about communication with some (by no means all) nursing students.

Although it is stating the obvious, you are more likely to get a response if, when leaving a voicemail message, you speak slowly and clearly, saying your first name, surname and cohort and explaining briefly why you are calling. If you want a reply, then give the number where you can be contacted by speaking slowly enough for it to be heard.

Nurse teacher comment

❝ As a teacher, it is difficult to hear a voicemail that says 'hello, it is Jo. It's urgent. Please ring me back on 020?XX?342?'. Jo who? What was that number? I have listened three times and more sometimes and still cannot catch it. On the student database I go through everyone called Jo (Josephine? Joe?). Then I try the numbers, and work out who it might be and discover the student moved house a month ago and has not told us. I do not want to sound grumpy, but please do say to your readers how important communicating with us is! ❞

Communication in clinical practice

During the course you will need to be able to speak with patients, clients and their families, fellow students and your mentors. Ideally you need to be able to write clearly as well, so that essays and reports, etc. are unambiguous. You will need to listen well in order to understand what is being said and where necessary pass messages accurately. You need to be succinct (i.e. keeping to the point and not rambling) and have a good understanding of 'professional' and nursing terminology. Chapter 11 explains more about this.

Learn to be aware of the tone, rhythm, pronunciation and speed of your speech. You will need to use professional language in exchanges with mentors and teachers. Later you may be required to *interpret* (i.e. to re-word) messages into everyday language to help your patient understand what is being said. When nursing people who do not have English as a first language, or others who have learning or sensory disability, non-verbal language, sign language and other alternative means of communication are helpful.

Basic tips to aid all communication

Communication is enhanced by facing the person you are speaking to, this can be seen in Figure 3.2. If they are sitting down you do the same; if they stand, so do you. If the person is hard of hearing, be aware of this. They may ask you to stand to one side (e.g. their best ear). Some eye contact is good, but not staring. Try always to wait for the other person to finish speaking without interruption. You can show you have listened by summarizing what they said to you, e.g. 'Ok, I will come back in an hour with a hot drink for you'.

Assertiveness

If you are going to be successful, you will have to get what you need to succeed. If you are shy or lacking in confidence, then learning some assertiveness skills could help. Back and Back (1991) say that when a person behaves assertively they express their needs in a direct and honest way. But, importantly, it is done in a manner that does not violate (disregard) the rights of others. By contrast, when a person behaves *aggressively* they ignore or dismiss the needs of others. Non-assertive people fail to stand up for their own rights and can be disregarded by others. Consider learning more about assertiveness if you feel it would help you.

Please read the following exercise imagining you are in this predicament.

Exercise 3.4

You are on a hectic SCBU (special care baby unit) that is short-staffed. Your mentor Jon is busy nursing a sick baby girl and also supporting her understandably anxious family. You are feeling worried because you need Jon to sign your practice assessment paperwork as soon as possible or you risk submitting it late at the university, at the end of the week. How can you possibly ask Jon to put your needs before the needs of others?

Please stop reading for a moment and think about how you might approach this difficult situation. Now read the following advice. How does it compare with what you had thought to say?

Your aim is to ask Jon for what you need in a clear and direct way.

It is not a good idea to open the conversation apologizing, e.g. 'Jon I am very sorry to bother you, I see you are busy, I hope you don't mind?'; this is not a good opening line.

Find time when you can get Jon's attention. Speaking steadily and calmly be direct: 'Jon, I need to speak with you sometime today please. It is about agreeing a time when we can meet so you can sign my assessment of practice document.'

Jon may agree a time with you at this point. If he does not, go on to give a reason for your request: 'Jon, it is very important that we plan a date to meet as my assessment is due in on Friday.'

Student comment

66 Ask for help if you need it. I have found all university lecturers to be really helpful when I have needed advice. Also, when out in placement, other students (who are further ahead) have also pointed me in the right direction, showing me how to present my portfolio or answering questions about bits of work that I was not sure about. I know there is a danger in asking other students but most of the people I have asked have been really good at telling me what I needed to know. When one student started to tell me what I should and should not put in a reflection, after I had spent hours completing it, I just smiled sweetly and ignored her. Learn how to use the advice given. 99

Saying 'no'

You may find yourself in a situation where you feel you are being asked to do something you would do not wish to. Saying 'no' can be hard. We worry people will not like us, or that they may be angry or hurt, or feel that we are unkind.

+...

Exercise 3.5

Marion, a fellow student, keeps suggesting you go with her for lunch, when really you would prefer to use the time in the library. Think of ways you could say 'no', and not hurt her feelings.

....

It would help here to keep your reply fairly short, but not abrupt. Avoid long explanations as to why you are saying no. It is important to be kind as you acknowledge the request made: 'Thank you for asking me Marion, but I need to go to the library now', is a direct, honest and clear response.

If she persists with the request, a sensitive and clear way to respond would be to say something like: 'It is thoughtful of you to ask me to join you, but I prefer to use my free time when I am here studying, so I can spend time with my family in the evenings.'

Negotiation

Skills in negotiation are needed when two or more people have conflicting needs. Sometimes you may need to negotiate with classmates or your mentor. The best negotiations end with a 'win/win' situation; where both parties feel that they obtained a satisfactory outcome. Important stages in negotiation are:

- Clarifying needs: be clear, direct and honest about what you need and why.
- Accepting needs: listen carefully, and value what the other person has to say: 'Ok, I accept that matters to you.' 'I see your need to do X'.
- Resolving needs: can be done by offering or asking for alternative suggestions—making agreements.

Values and beliefs: your own moral compass

The values and beliefs you have are important in your development as a nurse. If you value honesty, caring and kindness, and believe you should always do the best for patients and clients, and support your colleagues, by being a good team player, then you have a positive foundation on which to build. Know your weak spots and leave them at home!

Student comment

66 I found it hard when I was splitting up with my partner and feeling upset a lot of the time. Some days I just had to take a deep breath and push myself to go into my placement. It would have been so easy to stay in bed. But now I know it was the best thing to push myself. It was a hard lesson, but you have to put other people first. When you are on duty, that's what this job is about. (I am with a gorgeous new man now, so it all worked out in any case!) 99

Summary

You must look after yourself if you are going to be effective in your caring for other people and find the energy to do all that is expected of you on what is a demanding course. Support is available at all times and this chapter has introduced you to the main ways that this happens. Your success ultimately is down to you. Knowing and practicing the skills you need to succeed is important.

■ Top tips

- You and no one else is responsible for how well (or otherwise) you do on the programme.
- Who you are, and what you bring to the course, are important in determining your success.
- Being positive helps success.
- Communicate clearly—practice helps.
- Be assertive and clear in your interactions.
- Avoid compromising your success on the programme by doing too much additional paid work; budgeting helps.
- Make time to enjoy leisure pursuits and breaks.

■ Online resource centre

You can find further advice and practical tips to assure your time on the course goes well by going online to **www.oxfordtextbooks.co.uk/orc/hart/** where you can find useful checklists, exercises and online tools for financial and personal well being.

References

Back K and Back K (1991) *Assertiveness at work: a practical guide to handling awkward situations*, 2nd edn. McGraw Hill International, Maidenhead, Berkshire.

Davis M, Robbins Eshelman E and McKay M (2008) *The relaxation and stress reduction workbook*. New Harbinger publications, Oakland, California.

Eiser RJ and van der Pligt J (1988) *Attitudes and decisions*. Routledge, London.

National Union of Students (2008) **http://www.nus.org.uk/en/Student-Life/Money-And-Funding/The-true-cost-of-university**

Nursing and Midwifery Council (2008) *The code: standards of conduct, performance and ethics for nurses and midwives.* **http://www,nmc-uk.org/aArticle.aspx?ArticleD=3056**

Further reading

Kenworthy N, Snowley G and Gilling C (2001) *Common foundation studies in nursing*, 3rd edn. Churchill Livingstone, Edinburgh.

Lewis M (2005) *The money diet: the ultimate guide to shedding pounds off your bills and saving money on everything*, 2nd edn. Vermilion, London.

Websites

Martin Lewis, Money-saving expert: **www.moneysavingexpert.com**

NHS Choices website to support people who want to stop smoking cigarettes: **http://smokefree.nhs.uk/**

NHS Student Bursaries Home Page: **www.nhsstudentgrants.co.uk/**

Student Loan Company: **www.slc.co.uk**

Getting organized and managing your time

Sue Hart

The aims of this chapter are:

➤ To raise your awareness that good organization and time-management can help you to be successful

➤ To help you recognize the demands there can be on student nurses during the pre-registration programme

➤ To provide practical advice and guidance

➤ To suggest ways of creating a good environment for studying

Good organization and time-management skills will increase your chance of being successful on the pre-registration nursing programme. As long as it works for you, there is no 'right' or 'wrong' way of doing this. If being well-organized and keeping 'on top' of work comes naturally, you may already be thinking about how you will manage yourself throughout the course and it may be that you do not need the guidance that follows in this chapter. If, however, the reverse is true, please read on.

Student comment

❝ It was important simply to remember that support was there if needed, and to try to keep on top of the work you have to do, so that it doesn't get overwhelming. ❞

What follows contains simple, practical advice and suggestions about how you could organize yourself and manage your time on the course. There are comments from students and teachers, and several exercises you can do. The chapter has been included to encourage you to think about self-management and to give you some ideas about how this could be done. If you feel the ideas here are not helpful to you, then you must find your own way of getting organized. By not giving attention to these practicalities you may be risking your chances of success.

Nurse teacher comment *The basic tools of time-management and organization*

" Please make sure you have:

- A watch.
- An alarm clock, or one on a your mobile 'phone.
- A bag, big enough to hold an A4-sized file and books.
- A diary, minimum A5 size, as you will need to make multiple entries most days.
- A note book, a pocket dictionary and a pocket nurses' dictionary.
- Pens, highlighters (various colours) and pencils.
- A4 file paper. "

4.1 **Knowing yourself**

When preparing this chapter, we asked for comments from students about managing themselves and getting organized. The following shows the different approaches students take to managing themselves through the course, and shows how individual approaches vary.

Student comment

" I have found that I can keep up if I keep everything organized and get work done as soon as I can, even if the deadlines are some way off. You really have to stay on the ball, keep submission dates in your diary and a list of jobs to be done and prioritize. I would much rather have work done early, then, if a problem happens that takes up your time at home, you don't have to worry about trying to complete work at the last minute. This stood me in good stead during a time when my husband was in hospital and my time became very limited. "

" I've realized I am an 11th-hour girl. I can't seem to motivate myself till the last minute. I spent a lot of time worrying about that but now I've accepted that's the way I work best. So, from my perspective, we seem to have quite a long time to » complete the work, I've never felt it was too much in one go. Having said that, I have had to be more organized with my time-management, and keep on top of my 'domestic' jobs, so that when I have to drop everything to really knuckle down, I can. 99

66 It was difficult at first to get back into the learning environment, as I had left school at the age of 16, but I made a good friend on the first day and we've seen each other through some difficult times. Even though I am sponsored, I do have to work part-time too, but I have joined the bank staff, which enables me to take the time off when assignments are due in. Initially time-management was a problem, as I not only had a house to run, but work commitments too. The problems with time-management really begin when we are on placement, as often the shifts can be long days, therefore time off is for catching up on household duties (e.g. shopping) and possibly work too. To overcome this it is essential to organize yourself ahead of time, plan your work, and I *always* take my work with me to placement, as there can often be 10 minutes when you can get your books out and have a look at them, or write a few notes. It's amazing how these few minutes can make a difference. 99

Just like the students above, how you will need to organize yourself on a day-to-day basis will be personal to you and determined by your own circumstances. Please read below and see which of these personality stereotypes (if any) most closely resemble your thoughts about yourself.

+··

Exercise 4.1

Do you recognize yourself in any of these?

Fire fighter: you enjoy a crisis and the tasks pile up as you rush around.

Over-committer you never say no!

Aquarian you are very 'laid back'. Why do today what you can do tomorrow?

Chatty, chatty you socialize and shop and have fun before you do *anything* else.

Perfectionist you dot the 'I's and cross the 'T's; no rushed job can be good.

Worrier you tend to worry about everything. The idea that you could *enjoy* the course does not occur to you.

(See the online resource for more about personality types.)

Most likely none of the above 'fitted' you exactly, but it is possible that you recognized parts of yourself in some of them. To state the obvious, being a nursing student is part of your life now, but this is alongside the other roles you play in your life, e.g. sister, husband, partner, volunteer, athlete and friend.

Student comment

66 It helps to have a supportive family who understand the pressures on my time. 99

Please read through the 'personal inventory' below. Considering these points (and any others relevant to your own situation) can help give a feel for the demands on your time from others, how confident you feel and how much focus on time-management and self-organization you may need.

Exercise 4.2 Personal inventory

* What are the demands on your time from others? Do you have children, or do you have responsibilities as a carer for someone?
* Will you need to work part-time as well as studying?
* Do you think you will find the course difficult or are you confident already that you have the ability to succeed?
* What is your level of concentration, are you focused or easily distracted?
* How confident are you in your written work and numbers?
* Are you someone who can read a book chapter and retain information fairly effortlessly, or are you a slower reader, reliant on note-taking and frequent re-reading of sections?
* Do you consider yourself to be a well-organized and methodical person?
* Do you keep a diary (or other system of self organization) now and do you refer to it most days, or do you try to remember everything in your head?
* Do you feel you could you write an essay of 2500 words in two sittings?
* Do you often find it hard to start and complete tasks in time?
* Do you read for pleasure now?
* Have you just left school or just finished another course, pre-nursing, access or an NVQ, or is it many years since you were last in a classroom?
* In the past, did you start work on an assignment in your mind, or did you start on paper?
* Are you by nature a person who thinks steadily through tasks ahead, or do you prefer to start working on your assignment the day you are given the guidelines?
* Do you need the pressure of a deadline looming before doing any work?
* What time will you have to get up in order to be in time for an early shift for 7.00a.m. or in uni for 9.00a.m?
* How are you in the morning? Do you wake up ready to face the day or do you need time to 'come round'?

Hopefully, after the exercises you can think a bit more clearly about the sort of person you are, the demands there are on you and the likely impact on the programme for your time. At the start of the programme it also helps to think about *where* you are going to do the work. The next part of the chapter looks at creating an environment for your studying. Knowing yourself helps. If you are a 'morning person', then use these quiet hours to good effect. 'Larks' or morning people should avoid studying late at night, unless there is no alternative. Likewise, 'owls' may stay up long after others are sleeping and use time then.

4.2 Creating a good environment in which to study

To do well on the course you are going to need somewhere to study, to read, write and work at a computer. It will take some time and thought to make this happen. As the following shows, a little planning can make all the difference.

Imagine you are at home and it is winter, very cold outside. You plan an evening of relaxation for yourself. You find a TV film that starts in half an hour, just time to make some food. You make sure the room is warm, blinds drawn, mobile 'phone on silent, you plump up the cushions then settle yourself into an armchair, food on a tray (chocolate for afterwards) and switch on the television, in time to see the film start. What a great 'reward' for you after a busy day of looking after other people, a little self indulgence and escapism.

+ ....

Exercise 4.3

Please re-read the paragraph above noticing the *organization* that went into creating the ideal environment for your evening.

....

It took a few steps to turn an ordinary evening into something a bit more special. You allowed yourself not be disturbed, you ensured you were comfortable, well-fed and having 'researched' what was available on television, found a film you had wanted to see. An *unplanned* evening could have seen you 'fridge grazing' whatever you could find as you wandered in and out of your room half watching whatever channel was on the television at the time.

Now, to extend this idea, can you imagine creating a good environment for studying? Imagine you have an article that you must read in time for a discussion in class at 9.00a.m. tomorrow. The lecturer tends to direct questions to individuals, rather than the whole group.

This technique keeps everyone on their toes: you have *got* to get the reading done and you must do it well enough to sound plausible if asked a question. Where do you start? Just pick up the journal and read?

Student comment

❝ I have found it very difficult managing my time doing the theory work with a home and children, one being hyperactive. I have now found that if I can go somewhere quiet like the library a couple of days a week, it helps me keep on top of things and able to cope better and never put things off. ❞

It helps to think about creating the best possible environment for your studies. About an hour (or to be precise 50 minutes, the optimum time for studying without a break) in the right 'atmosphere' is at least equal to two hours of distracted, unfocused time. Considering the following may assist you in creating a good environment for studying.

Ideally, you need a *place of your own* to study, one that you can return to and find your papers undisturbed by others between your visits. If this place can also be home to your laptop or PC, then this would be even better. Finding such a place is easier if you live alone or in student accommodation; more difficult if you house- or room-share.

Nurse teacher comment

❝ If you live with others, suggest to them you all have some nights a week with no television or music for a couple of hours. Plan your reading evening when your flat-mate works late. If you have children, study when they are watching a DVD. Get your partner to bath the children, cook the supper. If you cannot get what you need at home, staying late in the library is an option. ❞

If possible, your study place will be quiet or one where you can get some undisturbed time. It must be warm in winter, well-ventilated in the summer and have a desk, a comfortable desk chair (adjustable with arms would be perfect) good enough light, somewhere to store your work and a clock. To complete the reading in time for tomorrow, you need to give yourself enough *time* to do it. This means focused, concentration time. With no distractions, you are going to work much more efficiently.

Studying in groups

Some students prefer to study alone. Others choose to study in pairs or even in a small group. Whilst plagiarism (copying the work of others) is unacceptable (see Chapter 5), working together, sharing thoughts (e.g. about what you are reading) and supporting each other can be very helpful and an important part of the course. With planning, you could have agreed with friends to have all read the article for tomorrow's lecture by a given date, then talk through your understanding of it one lunch-time before the lecture.

? Stop and think

Be nice to yourself when you are studying. Have enough breaks and give yourself treats, drink and eat enough and then later celebrate your achievement. After a whole day writing an assignment, you deserve to relax.

It is up to you to create the best environment you can for studying in, hopefully at home, where you can feel relaxed and comfortable. If this is impossible, then find out if your department has study suites or quiet rooms; the university library will have such rooms. Most libraries have extended opening hours to suit both 'larks' and 'owls'. It is wise to use your time well. Half an hour spent reading in the library at lunch-time may mean half an hour less reading at home when you would rather be spending time with your partner or friends.

4.3 Organizing your time

Student comment

❝ I find that I have to plan well in advance, by looking at the timetable for the module, because it is not a regular timetable when you are in the same times each week. I find it hard just to remember what lectures we have coming up and what reading/research/tasks I have to complete in time. I have a copy of the timetable on the wall behind my desk and have also made my own 'yearly' planner, with all the months and dates on. I mark on this using a colour coding system, when I have to have tasks or assignments completed by—that way I can see exactly how much time I have left to complete that particular task. ❞

+··

Exercise 4.4

Does time-management need to be difficult? Think about the following:

You know how much time something will take to complete,

You put aside the time, and then

You *use the time* to do whatever is needed,

Hey presto! You complete the task on time.

··

Although the statement above is *logical*, it fails to consider any factors that may interfere with progress towards completion of a task. Also, in reality, it is not always possible to say how long an assignment will take. Overestimating the time is less of a problem than the reverse, as at least you give yourself time to complete. Underestimating how long an assignment may take can lead to last-minute panic as a deadline draws closer. In such circumstances it is unlikely that your best work is produced. One way to get over these problems is to know yourself and the demands on you (as discussed above) and to pay attention to how you manage your time. To help focus on this think…

Diary, dates and deadlines!

Diary

Missing the deadline for submitting an assignment or being late for class is avoidable. Furthermore, it is in your *best interests* to avoid such situations, as it can give your teachers and mentors the impression that you are not yet developing professionally. For obvious reasons this is not good. (See more about professional behaviour in Chapter 14.) One simple way to avoid such mishaps is to develop good diary-keeping habits.

We recommend a diary of at least A5 size with a week per view format (see Figure 4.1). These usually have a year planner as well.

Dates

As soon as the following information is available, put in your diary:

- The date, start time and location of *all* your lectures and seminars, groups and other uni activities.
- Any other meetings, e.g. occupational health, personal tutor.
- Examination dates and submission dates for course work in red.
- A '2 weeks to submission date or examination' reminder for yourself.
- Your start and finish dates and times each day when in placement.
- The dates for your assessment in practice in red.

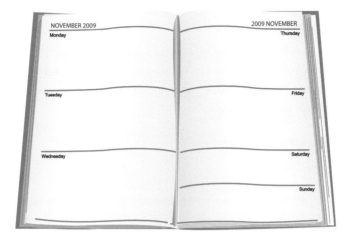

Figure 4.1 A5 diary

- A single diagonal line through holiday days.
- Remember to fill in your personal commitments (nights out, dentist, dog to vet).

Keep all your information in the one diary: running two diaries does not work.

+···

Exercise 4.5

Make yourself an A4-sized printout of your course flow (see Chapter 2 about course flows). Then you could fold this in half and securely attach it to the back of your diary.

···

If this system is going to work you will need to make it your habit to carry your diary almost all the time. Imagine your friends suggest a day trip to the coast on a Sunday a few weeks ahead. You agree and promise you will drive in your car. Later you realize that you have committed yourself the day before your next assignment is due in. If you had been able to look at your diary, you could have avoided this. Get used to picking your diary up as you do your mobile 'phone and keys.

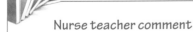

Nurse teacher comment

❝ I do realize that some people nowadays prefer to use electronic palm-held diaries, the diary on a mobile 'phone, a blackberry or a computer diary such as a calendar. These are all useful in their way. However, for *practical* purposes when on a course such as this, an old-fashioned paper diary is best. It is mobile, you can write in it easily, it does not run out of battery at an awkward time and you do not have to switch it off in lectures (like you would a mobile 'phone diary!). ❞

Deadlines (1): backward planning

Imagine you have to write a 1500-word assignment due in on October 15th. Based on your honest self-analysis from the exercises in 'Knowing yourself' above, estimate the time you will need to complete the task. Check that both the deadline date and the '2 weeks to submission' reminder are in your diary.

- Deadline Oct 15th
- Reminder Oct 1st

You estimate you will need at least three evenings for background reading and note-taking, and 2 days for writing. Scan your diary to find available time between today and the '2 weeks to go reminder' date, and note in your diary when you will do the work for this assignment. If you have not yet searched for the books and articles you will need for this, also find time in your diary to go to the library.

Using this *backward planning* method, your work should be finished 2 weeks before it is due in. If, when writing an assignment, you factor in time for a delay (e.g. wanting to visit your grandmother who unexpectedly has been taken into hospital), it need not be a disaster. With this method, if you lose some of your planned time, then you still have a chance of recovering the situation and submitting on the due date. If all has gone well and you manage to finish as you originally planned, then submit your work as soon as the university rules permit, ahead of the deadline. Then either enjoy some time between assignments, or start working on your next task.

In any eventuality you are advised always to submit your work 24 hours (or more) ahead of schedule. With a 10.00a.m. deadline, it takes only a traffic jam, a delayed train or a printer breakdown *that morning*, to prevent you handing in on time. Why chance it?

Deadlines (2): big elephants and little elephants

This is a useful technique, particularly when you have several deadlines that are all still some way off. Imagine it is October. You have to complete an end-of-first-year project for which you have already been given the guidelines. It is due in on June 7th.

In the autumn months the elephant is small, you can see it far off in the distance. Steadily working, keeping 'on track', is helping you to progress. By January the elephant will be much bigger, by April bigger still. The weeks before the final deadline it will be big, the last days huge, in the room with you (see Figure 4.2)! How you feel about the elephant then, will depend on how well you have planned, organized and managed your time. If you have let progress slip, it is likely you will feel stressed, the elephant will feel menacing. If you are on course with your work, the elephant will still be big, but standing quietly in the corner of the room, present but not threatening. And you will be ready to submit.

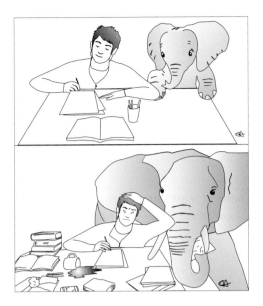

Figure 4.2 Big elephants and little elephants. Artist: Emma Heaton

4.4 **Priorities**

With many competing demands, e.g. an assignment to finish, reading to do, personal tutor to see, lecture to attend… as the saying goes, it sometimes can be 'hard to see the wood for the trees'. How do you work out what is your priority? Figure 4.3 is a simple tool to help you decide.

On any given day something may be urgent, other things important, yet others in the back of your mind as something to be getting on with next week. An extract from your diary may look like Figure 4.4.

Submitting your essay is a priority *that day*, urgent = 25

The enquiry-based learning (EBL) is due within 2 days, very important = 16

The journal article must be read by next Monday = 2

Remember, day by day your priorities change. At 10.00a.m. (plus 1 second) on Monday October 22nd the deadline for submitting the essay has passed. Getting it in on time was a 25-point priority. By Monday October 29th, being prepared for your seminar becomes a 25-point priority.

This technique helps you to think about your priorities on any given day. Once you get used to thinking like this, it should become second nature.

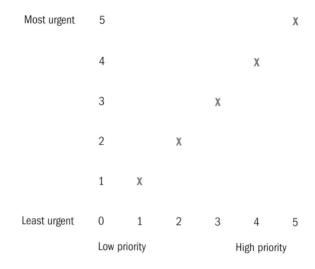

Most urgent   5   X

               4   X

               3   X

               2   X

               1   X

Least urgent   0   1   2   3   4   5

               Low priority   High priority

Scoring
Urgent and high priority = 25 (i.e. 5x5)
Medium to high priority = 16
Medium priority = 9
Low to medium priority = 4
Least urgent and low priority = 2

Figure 4.3 The relationship between urgency and priority

Monday 22nd October: (Uni)

10.00   (at latest)   submit Foundations of nursing care essay (*submit by 9.30 or may be late for lecture*)

10.00   Lecture (bio science – Lecture theatre D2, lecture theatre block)

Library after lunch; re article for seminar

13.00   Personal tutor group (Nursing Department, level 3 room 14)

14.00   Self directed work: Library time – work on enquiry based learning presentation for Wednesday 24th

15.00   Meet group re timetable for Wednesday visit to practice (Union coffee bar)

Evening: Read journal articles for seminar next Monday 29th 11.00.

Figure 4.4 Nursing student's diary extract

> ••• **A word about** Saving time—work straight on to your computer
>
> This can save hours of time. Learning to use the 'cut and paste' facility is a must. Also *save your work regularly*. A useful trick: from time to time as you are writing, send an email to yourself with your work as an attachment. In Microsoft Word, click on 'File', on the drop-down menu click on 'Send to', then click on 'Mail recipient as an attachment' and send. If you put your own email address in your 'address book' it makes this process even quicker; about 8 seconds. That is not long to keep your work safe. It is easy to delete the email copies if you do not need them.

4.5 **Organizing your paperwork**

If you are a naturally organized person, the following will be perfectly logical to you, so skip this section. If you struggle to get organized, then this should help.

> **Nurse teacher comment**
>
> 66 When you feel you are drowning in new information, and as teachers we do accept that nursing students experience this sensation sometimes, your instincts may be to bin the lot. Please resist this temptation. The simple truth is that there is a lot you need to know and reading, filing and re-visiting important information is essential throughout the programme. 99

There is no easy way to say this: expect to receive a lot of information from your first day and throughout your first year. This may be on paper, via electronic means (email, blogs, and web-sites), on notice-boards or by word of mouth in a lecture or seminar. You will come to learn that often nurse teachers like to tell you things and then be reassured that you know what they have told you by making the information available to you by one of the above means. This 'belt and braces' approach is adopted in part to embed your learning and understanding, and also so that there is evidence that you were given the necessary information that you needed to have. What you then do with the information you are given is the $64,000 question.

Good habits

Developing effective *filing, storing and information retrieval habits* will be invaluable. Why? Please consider the following:

- If the information you have been given was not important, the staff would not waste time creating the document and making it available to you.

- A handout that does not seem relevant to you now, *will* be relevant in the future, or you would not have been given it.

- Having to ask for a replacement copy of something you were given is time-consuming for both you and the staff, and adds to costs, so is not welcome.

You are advised to keep every piece of paper you are given from day one of the programme until the end and to adopt a system like the one that follows to ensure you can find it again when you need it.

How you can manage your paper work?

Like *diary, dates and deadlines!* There are three key steps:

- create files

- label files and

- divide files.

Creating files (or folders or binders)

Student comment

❝ Folders! Make sure you file your class notes in order. I have a separate folder for A&P, biosciences and then an additional one for the modules I am studying. This works for me but some have different systems. Find what works for you. ❞

First, what you need: buy some A4 ring binders or arch lever files, some A4-size dividers, an A4 hole-punch and packs of A4 file paper with lines and margins. If you do not have the money to buy the files you can, almost as effectively, use clearly labelled cardboard files or even cardboard boxes and sheets of coloured paper as dividers. Label the file (or ring binder or box) with its name on the outside and also label your dividers (more about this below).

Now, what to do: on every piece of paper (or on sets of papers stapled or clipped together) note down in the top right-hand corner information you may need in the future. For example, the date when you were given the paper and the name of the person who gave it to you.

- For the paper *you* generate, e.g. notes you have taken in class, write the date, the title of the session and the name of the teacher who delivered the lecture.

- For a printed document sourced on the internet you could simply highlight the date and the website address where it appears on the paper.

- Then file the paper in (a) the *correct* ring binder/file and (b) in the correct division.

! **Fact box**

There are some excellent stationery deals online for individual buyers; ever better ones for bulk purchases. If a group of you get together to do this, you will get more for your money than in the high street stores.

Labelling and dividing files

If the above system is going to work, then organizing the files, the labelling and dividing have to be effective to do the job. One approach you could use is to think of the three key skills sets we have mentioned several times already: 'theory', 'practice' and 'professional'. Everything you are given or that you create should fall into one (or sometimes more than one) of these categories. So a good starting point would be to organize your ring binders or files under each of these headings.

A 'theory file' could be created for each theory module or unit in the first year. You could create this at the beginning of the programme, as you will know by then the names of all your year-one theory modules (see your programme handbook or information on your department's student website). Use *dividers* to further separate the file into sections containing the paper work you were (a) given in class (by the lecturer) or (b) notes that you made yourself during the lecture or seminar.

Further information to be filed, with the dividers clearly labelled could include:

- Information regarding the assignment for the module.
- The module reading list.
- Module seminar or enquiry-based learning topics.
- Your instructions for preparing and presenting enquiry-based learning work or a seminar.
- Instructions/guidelines for any self-directed work.
- Notes you have made when doing the general background reading for the module.
- Notes you have made in readiness for writing the module assignment.
- Useful information for the module that you have decided to download and print from your PC.
- Any journal articles.
- List of useful references.
- The contact details of teachers leading the module.
- Anything else relevant to the module not easily categorized using the headings above could be placed in a 'miscellaneous' division at the back.

Files for your practice information

You could develop these in a variety of different ways, but one for each placement is ideal. As soon as you know where you are going, label the outside of the file with the placement name and note on a sheet of paper to go inside the details, as in Figure 4.5. (We have put templates for this information in the online resource centre.) If any details change (e.g. if your mentor is unwell and is replaced by someone else), remember to make the correction. Carefully recording this information is very important to you with regards to the 'sign-off mentor' system (see Chapter 13).

Suggested *dividers in your practice* file could be as follows:

- Information given to you by your mentor.
- Any particular instructions issued by the university with regard to your practice.
- Material you are gathering for your **portfolio** and any practice-based assignments or reflections (see Chapter 12).
- Journal articles or downloaded material relevant to the practice area.
- A record of your dates and hours in practice.

Placement: Second placement, year one, child

Dates in placement: 04/04/10 – 16/05/10

Location: Holly Unit, St Andrew's Hospital

Type of placement: Special Care Baby Unit

Telephone number: xxxxx xxxxxx

Mentor: Staff nurse Mike Smith,

Associate/co mentor: Nurse Alexis Nyoni

Mentor phone number: xxxxx xxxxxx

Email address of mentor: m.smith@hollyunit.standrews.nhs.org.uk

Nurse in Charge: Sister Vicky Brampton

University link teacher: Jean Perkins

Figure 4.5 Placement information proforma

- A record of any sickness or absence you had and, if applicable, the dates when you made up the hours.

- A note carried over from your previous placement with regard to hours missed and consequently needing to be made up in *this* placement.

Your 'professional file' can be the place where you keep all the information you are given or you create yourself with regard to the *professional development* aspect of the course. The NMC booklets you have been given could be filed here, as could information about your 'home' NHS Trust, such as transportation between sites, uniform policy, infection control policy, and health and safety advice.

But surely paperwork could easily fit into one or more folders?

Yes. You will occasionally have paperwork that could go equally well into any of your files. An example could be a paper about the 'management of consent to treatment when working with patients who have a learning disability in acute hospital settings'. The *management of consent* is a *professional* issue, in this context relating to practice in an acute care setting. In such a circumstance, simply make your decision, place the article in one file and in the other put a tracer note to yourself. This could simply be a piece of file paper in your professional file that says: 'see paper re consent' in clinical practice file, under acute care setting/surgery.

4.6 **Organizing your computer**

How to manage electronic information

With electronic information you need to decide first if the document needs to be turned into a hard (paper) copy. For example, your personal tutor may send you something by email and suggest you print it out and keep for your records. If necessary, print it out and file as with 'paper' above.

X **Avoid** Making unnecessary hard copies

Considering the costs (environmental and financial) and the volume of information you are dealing with, the less printing you have to do the better. Getting used to reading from the screen of your PC or laptop can take time, but the information there is just as good as on paper. Unless it is a 'read-only' document (which you cannot change) you can you make notes on it. Using a bright colour to do this can be effective.

Organizing information that you want to keep in an electronic format follows the same principles as above. All word processing programmes have a system for organizing files. Create electronic files (with names and sub-files for divisions) in just the same way as suggested for paper. If you are not yet confident when using a computer, it may help you to understand that file management, such as that described above, is a very basic activity, and one that you are advised to learn as soon as possible, and certainly before you start receiving a lot of information. You could ask the staff in your university IT department if they could help you. They may have a handout or online training-package already developed to help students to manage and organize files and folders. Some students struggle with IT skills, so nurse teachers will ensure this topic is covered during teaching time (e.g. a lecture on IT) or by directing students to introductory e-learning tools. If the uni have not addressed this and you have a need, they may provide something if a group of students get together to ask. If not, this is more likely to be included for you if there are a few of you who need this training, so ask around for others who would benefit. You could also buy (or find a library book) to go through the basics of file management for the system you are using.

• • • **A word about** 'Backing-up' files on your computer

Students who are inexperienced with 'e-working' sometimes worry about 'losing everything'. It helps to know that there are techniques to 'back up' (make safe) your files and documents. It is simply a question of knowing what and how. You can copy work to memory sticks, a re-write CD or even on to 'floppy discs', but only the latter if your computer is quite old. Also see the tip about emailing your work to yourself above.

! **Fact box** 'To do' lists

These can be helpful to note all you need to do in an allotted time. It helps keep you focused and provides a sense of achievement as you strike through the completed actions. It can be a useful short-term measure for getting things done.

Summary

Good organization can minimize the extent to which you will find the course stressful and demanding, because you will feel 'on top' of it. Knowing yourself also helps you to recognize the demands on you and your own patterns of time-wasting; when you see them coming, you can stop them before they interfere with your work. Try to balance perfectionism with being *realistic* about what is expected of you and what you can expect of yourself. You will pass the course well if you get average marks in everything. Getting high marks for an essay is satisfying, but if this comes at the cost of failing another piece of work, it loses its shine. Remember that part of the challenge you are being set is to do the work in the time allocated. Teach your self good habits (carrying a journal to read, a note book and your diary). Use your time well. Recognize that personal effectiveness and self-management are important features in the developing professional; you are acquiring skills that you will need to be successful in your career.

■ Top tips

- Getting organized is a must. It does not matter how you do it, as long as you develop a system that works for you.
- Always refer to any guidelines that the university gives you, with regard to written work (more in Part 2 about this).
- Never rely on hearsay for important information, such as the change of a submission date. Teachers will ensure you know 'officially' if this is the case.
- Always plan your work time with your deadline and '2 weeks to go reminder' in mind.
- Plan time *in your diary* to research, and write in the same way that you would put another event in your diary.
- Always keep a text book or journal in your bag—you never know when you will have time to read.
- Use the time you have set aside to read, to read!
- Use time well. Read for 20 minutes on your home-to-uni bus journey every day and you will have read for over three and a half hours in one week.
- Know what *you* need to do to succeed. This may be different to others; do not compare yourself.
- Understand the concept of 'good enough'. Do not focus so much on getting one piece of work perfect, that you lose time to do the others.
- From time to time you may need to revive your flagging motivation. Expect the dips. Talk to your personal tutor or friends. Remind yourself why you came to the course and that one day soon you will be a registered nurse.

■ Online resource centre

 To make the most of the organisation skills in this chapter, now go online to www.oxfordtextbooks.co.uk/orc/hart/ to download useful templates and read tips that can save you a lot of time in the future.

■ Further reading

Evans C (2008) *Time-management for dummies*. John Wiley and Sons, New Jersey.

Forster M (2000) *Get everything done and still have time to play*. Hodder & Stoughton, London.

Mitchell A (2007) *Time-management for manic mums*. Hay House, London.

PART 2

Getting through!

Learning in a university

Sue Hart

The aims of this chapter are:

➤ To understand how you learn

➤ To understand the role of an 'adult learner'

➤ To be introduced to some of the methods of teaching and learning at university

➤ To introduce referencing

This chapter will help you understand *how you learn* as an individual, and explain the *culture of learning and teaching* in higher education. It will help you to be successful if you can recognize how university learning differs from that at school and in further education colleges, and adapt to this. This chapter introduces *academic progression;* meaning how you progress from one academic level to the next. It will show how your course will gradually become more demanding as you work your way from year one to the end.

5.1 The culture of teaching and learning in a university

Nurse lecturers use various teaching and learning methods to ensure students attain the required knowledge, understand the academic subjects and appreciate the cultural and ethical issues necessary to fulfil the requirements for professional registration. University learning is different from learning at school and from the NVQ learning you may have done at college. In university you are an adult learner. This refers both to the relationship that you will have with the people who are teaching you and supporting your learning, and how you learn.

At school, and especially when teaching young children, teachers are responsible for making all the decisions about what is learned, and how and when it is learned. At school the tendency is to see the teacher as a 'font of knowledge' imparting information and facts, with pupils passively accepting what is taught, without necessarily questioning if it is true or correct.

Adults learning at university

The work of Malcolm Knowles (1984) is helpful in explaining the *culture of university learning*. Knowles developed the concept of *andragogy*, also referred to as *the art and science of teaching adults*. He argues that adult learners need to know why they are learning what they are learning and to understanding that the learning is relevant for their needs. In adult learning settings, the previous experiences and the knowledge and understanding of learners is taken into consideration by those who are teaching. This is because most adult learners have experience and knowledge that can be used as a learning resource. Also, adults are expected to be self-motivated, to learn for their own self-satisfaction and for 'real-life benefits' (e.g. to become a registered nurse).

An adult relationship with lecturers is intended to be more of an equal one than with teachers at school. Adult learners in universities are not dependent on their teachers as are pupils. As an adult learner you will:

- Decide how much (or little) work you do. Whether you apply yourself diligently or do the minimum and risk failing, is your choice.

- Be given deadlines to submit assessments. If you fail to submit on time you must live with the consequences.

- Not be 'chased' by teachers to produce work.

- You will be expected to be self-directing, and take responsibility for a significant amount of your own learning.

- Often be 'guided' to learn rather than 'taught', although with certain methods of teaching (such as lectures) you will be given information rather than necessarily interacting with the lecturer

Adult learning behaviour

 Avoid Disturbing the lecture

In all settings at university you must ensure that your mobile phone is turned off, as this can be distracting to fellow students and the lecturer, as well as diverting your attention from what is being said.

In such a culture students are (obviously) expected to behave as an adult, taking responsibility for their own learning, being punctual, courteous, reliable and committed to the course and attentive in class. In other words, adult learners do everything they can to engage in learning, respecting lecturers and other members of the support staff who are there to help.

Adult learners also understand the responsibility they have to their fellow students. When in lectures, adult learners do all they can to support their peers, to listen when they speak or answer a question, and to avoid causing any disruption that may affect the learning or concentration of others.

5.2 **Understanding the way that you learn**

We have said that the way you learn at university is different from school, but how? There are numerous *theories of learning* but all seem to agree that learning involves change. Bloom's Taxonomy (1956) is just one of many ways that learning can be explained. 'Taxonomy' simply means a way of classifying or categorizing something. Understanding Bloom's approach will help you appreciate how your learning on the pre-registration nursing course is structured and assessed.

Bloom's taxonomy is divided into three parts or 'domains'. These are:

The cognitive domain, which deals with *knowledge and thinking.*

The psychomotor domain, which deals with *skills.*

The affective domain, which deals with attitudes, e.g. *feelings and emotions.*

Please look at Table 5.1. Note how each 'domain' (cognitive, psychomotor and affective) is subdivided and ordered in degrees of difficulty. As a learner you must master the simple before moving onto the more complex areas. This could be likened to a computer game where you have to complete each level before moving onto the next.

To be successful in the first year of your course *at a minimum*, you will be expected through completion of your assessments, to demonstrate you have achieved progress along the continuum in the domain skills in purple (non-bold). How quickly and well you progress will depend on your previous experience and educational achievements, your confidence and the learning opportunities open to you. It could be expected, for example, that Masters or 'fast-track students' with previous degrees would progress towards the complex skills much more quickly, although this may not be the case. However, to be performing at the levels

---

! **Fact box**

You will become familiar with the words 'knowledge', 'skills' and 'attitudes'. They will feature in your assessment of practice and in learning outcomes for your modules.

Domain	Concerned with	Moving from the simple to the more complex					
Cognitive	Knowledge	Recall data	Understand	**Apply**	**Analyse**	**Synthesis**	Evaluation
Psychomotor	Skills	Copy	Follow instructions	**Develop precision**	**Combine related skills**	**Become expert**	
Affective	Attitude	Awareness	React	**Value**	**Organise**	**Adopt behaviour**	

Table 5.1 Anticipated student nurse journey of development in the first year (adapted from the work of Bloom 1956).

highlighted purple (non-bold) by the end of year one, will give you a solid foundation for your move to the second year. To have progressed to achieve any outcomes to the right of the box, highlighted in dark purple bold will be a bonus. (If you look at the grading criteria examples across the programme at the online resource, you will see in detail how it is the practice for lecturers to award more marks for assessments that demonstrate the more complex skills.) Read Chapter 6 for more information.

> ••• **A word about** Marking guidelines
>
> For example, at level 4 (formerly level 1) between 40 and 49% marks may be awarded for work that shows 'adequate knowledge and understanding', but has 'mainly descriptive use of knowledge' with 'little evidence used'.
>
> However, 70–79% are given if the assessment shows a 'very good level of knowledge and understanding' and has a 'very good use of relevant literature from a range of disciplines'. (Extract from a level 4 marking guideline—see online resource.)

The following explains development across the programme in each domain

- As you move from left to right along the cognitive domain you are expected to acquire knowledge (through attending lectures and reading), and be expected to recall data (such as in an exam or test) to show that you understand.

- When a nurse in practice performs a nursing activity (such as the removal of sutures/stitches) s/he is doing this by using psychomotor skills. As a novice, just beginning in the development of your nursing skills practise, you first must learn by observing and then copying, and following instructions.

- The affective domain can be explained by thinking about what you bring to your work, both personally and professionally. It is about how you are in you role. Your attitude as a nurse is very important (are you considerate in your dealings with patients and clients?). Are you alert, aware, observing and anticipating needs (such as noticing a patient is upset and needs to talk) and will you react by responding to them?

The skills in dark purple bold in Table 5.1 are those that you will be expected to acquire during the later part of the programme. For example, to become a registered nurse you must be able to *apply* the knowledge you have to the practice setting, and be able to *analyse* information, e.g. by weighing up the information given to you and making judgements.

Academically more able students (such as those on M-level courses) should also develop the even more complex skills of *synthesis*, i.e. an ability beyond analysis, to combine a number of variables or concepts into a coherent whole (see Oxford University Press, Dictionary 2003) and *evaluation,* that is assessing the value of something (e.g. evaluating how well a new care-planning system is meeting the needs of patients in your unit).

Bloom's theory is helpful as it shows how learners progress by learning that which is easily achievable and later that which is less so. The development of *your* skills will depend on how quickly you learn. It is important to remember that the course is not a competition, nor is it a race. You are an adult learner with your own learning style. You may learn quickly in some areas and slowly in others. If you have a specific learning need (e.g. dyslexia) this may mean you need to take longer to do your written work and reading. However, you may well learn rapidly in practice.

Learning styles

Student comment

❝ Try not to force yourself into a working or learning style that may not suit you; just because a method works for your friend, does not mean that it is right for you. ❞

Chapter 4 highlighted that self-organization and time-management needs are personal to the individual. What follows shows that *how we learn what we learn* is also personal to us. We all have our own learning style (referred to above) and understanding this, and using it, can help a student be successful. For this the work of Honey and Mumford (1992) is informative. They differentiate between the following learning styles:

- Activist   (learn by doing)
- Theorist   (need to know the models/theories behind the action)
- Pragmatist   (like to apply their learning to practice)
- Reflector   (like to observe and think about their learning)

See the online resource for more information about these and to assess your own learning style.

5.3 Academic progression

This term is used to show how the pre-registration nursing course, and other courses at university, become more challenging and demanding for learners as they progress. Table 5.2 shows the standard progression through the academic levels from 4 to 8 and the award given on successful completion of each stage.

It is usual that the first year of a pre-registration nursing programme is at academic level 4 (formerly level 1 in England). If you are studying for a diploma in nursing, usually you will be taught at level 5 (formerly level 2) for the second 2 years. Alternatively, if you are studying for a higher diploma, an ordinary or honours degree, you will be required to study at level 6 for at least part of the final year. Masters students study at level 7. *Exactly how much of the time is spent studying at the different levels will be particular to your own university, as there are no set national rules guiding such matters.* (See the online resource.)

Level 4 Certificate	This is equivalent to the first year of study on a university course. In order to progress to level 5, you need 120 credits at this level or the equivalent. Need to demonstrate knowledge and understanding at a basic level. Work mainly descriptive.
Level 5 Diploma	This is the undergraduate diploma level. It is equivalent to the second year of a university degree course. To be awarded a diploma you need to have 120 credits at level 5 (plus 120 from level 4). Work more discursive than level one, with some analysis required.
Level 6 Degree	This is degree level. To gain an honours degree you need 120 credits at level 6 (plus 240 from previous levels). Most nursing degree programmes will have compulsory core modules such as evidence based practice or research methods. Studying at level 6 means there is more in-depth analysis and critique of evidence than required at diploma level.
Post-graduate certificate or diploma	This is an interim point between degree and Master's level qualification. These are exit points for learners who do not want to do a full Masters dissertation but have studied at level 7 or M Level.
Level 7 Masters degree	In order to access this level you need to have completed Level 6 study or as a post-graduate nurse show through other learning that you are capable of study at this level. Masters level study incorporates application of research and the assimilation of new ideas. Masters degrees require a dissertation, which is an extended piece of work that can be either research or literature based.
Level 8 MPhil and PhD or Professional Doctorate	Study at this level is research based and at doctoral level it is about originality and in the case of professional doctorate, about extending the boundaries of your professional practice.

Table 5.2 Showing progression through academic levels, adapted from **http://www.wipp.nhs.uk/tools_gpn/toolu4_academic_of_study.php**.

Year One			
Module	Level	Credits	Assessment
1. Essential Nursing Skills	4	20	Essay on care planning, 1500 words (50%). Online drug calculation exam 1 hour (50%)
2. Health & Social Care in Society	4	40	1 x 3hour known topic exam based on a scenario.
3. Practice Module	4	60	Portfolio of Practice Evidence/ Assessment by mentor in practice (50%). 2,000 word case study (50%).

Table 5.3 Example of assessments in a year one nursing programme.

Academic credits

You will note that Table 5.2 refers to *credits*. ('In order to progress to level 5, you need 120 *credits*' at level 4.) The *academic credit rating* for a module (sometimes called CAT points) is dependent on the amount of work required to complete the module assessment. This is not consistent across all universities. All 'theory' modules will have a credit rating attached to them and, if your course has 'practice' modules, meaning that your time in placement is also organized into modules; these too will have a credit rating.

How the modules are organized will vary from university to university. See Table 5.3 for an example of what assessment, level and credit ratings may look like in a year one nursing programme.

In this example there are two theory modules, Essential Nursing Skills and Health and Social Care in Society, and one Practice module. Each has a credit rating. On successful completion of the Essential Nursing Skills module a student would be awarded 20 credits at Level 4. Success in the following two modules would mean being awarded a further 100 credits, meaning a total of 120 credits in year one. *In all universities, to successfully complete the first year you must have at least 120 credits at level 4.*

+···

Exercise 5.1

Find out the module titles, credit levels and assessment requirements for *all* of the first year of your programme. This information will be in your programme handbook or on the department website.

Plan a work schedule (following the advice in Chapter 4). Remember, the amount of work involved in a 20-credit module will differ from one worth 40 credits.

···

5.4 **Teaching and learning at university**

Methods

These can be divided into those that are led by lecturers and those that are mainly student-led, or a combination of both. When teaching and learning are lecturer-led, the teacher, for the most part, transmits ideas and information, e.g. in a lecture. In contrast, student-led learning is where you, the student, discover things for yourself. Sometimes students may be asked to present their findings to the rest of the class, e.g. in a method of learning called enquiry-based learning (EBL) or problem-based learning (PBL). Finally, sharing between the two methods allows the knowledge and experience of all (lecturers and students) to contribute to the experience, e.g. in a discussion group or seminar. Table 5.4 shows some of the more common teaching and learning activities in use and your role as a student in each. It also overviews some teaching and learning methods and the student's role in them.

Lecture: Lectures are usually formal presentations. You are expected to listen in silence to the lecturer and take notes. In an *interactive lecture* the teachers will ask for your contribution, usually by posing questions. Some universities have the facility to allow students to respond with keypads when the lecturer poses a question with different possible answers.

Small group work: Sometimes a lecturer may split a class into small groups, enabling each to focus on a different aspect of a question. Often these classes end with 'feedback' from each group. This adds to the knowledge and understanding of all. You are expected to participate in the activity, drawing on your experience of practice so far, and listening to the experiences of others.

Seminar: Seminar groups usually follow lectures and are used to clarify and develop the points made there. Sometimes lecturers give students directed reading to complete before the seminar. Occasionally seminars are student led. Here students are required to summarise an article they have been asked to read to stimulate discussion.

Workshops: If you see the term 'workshop' you should expect it to be an interactive event. It may be a whole day event to explore a particular subject – e.g. 'vulnerable people'. Workshops usually consist of a variety of teaching and learning methods. It might start with a mini lecture, group work, then self directed learning, and presentations at the end. You are expected to participate in the group activities and be responsible for finding out what you need to know.

Enquiry or problem based inquiry or learning [EBL. PBI or PBL] With guidance from your lecturers this activity aims to get you to learn in small groups about problems, needs and issues relevant to your practice. You are given the choice of topics or a patient/client scenario as a *trigger* to prompt your thinking. Your task is then to search for information to present back to the larger group. How you present the information is usually up to your group. Be innovative and creative. Do role plays, develop an interactive quiz, or make a movie…

Role play Imagine you need to learn about working within a budget. This could be taught in a lecture. Alternatively your group could be given an imaginary budget and be asked to *role play* (that is to act, get a feel for what it is like) being an accountant or health care professional with a list of patients with a variety of needs requiring costly treatment. In the relative comfort of a classroom you could experience what it may be like to make such decisions *for real*. You must play the role needed in order for this learning to be effective.

Some of the topics you will need to learn are best taught by **demonstration** once you have had the necessary theory background. For example, you will need to learn correct hand washing techniques. Once demonstrated you may be expected to practise the skill.

Simulation Imagine you need to learn how to resuscitate a patient. This cannot be done safely on a living person, so a model or a mannequin (whole body) model is used. Alternatively, a smaller model representing a part of the anatomy may be used, e.g. a nose to learn how to pass a nasogastric tube.

Table 5.4 Examples of teaching and learning methods used in universities.

+

Exercise 5.2

Think about the different sessions you have had so far on the course. What do you like or dislike about each of them? Are you making the most of your e-learning opportunities? What are some of the advantages and disadvantages of this type of learning?

Electronic learning/virtual learning environments (VLEs)

This is a growing phenomenon and is definitely the future! Universities everywhere are now using e-learning tools. The following are some of the ones used. Some universities develop their own e-learning systems. If so, you will be guided to that resource. Web-based technology can easily be accessed on and off campus (24/7). You can work alone or interact with classmates.

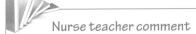

Nurse teacher comment

66 We use a lot of web-based learning materials and students are expected to download these and makes notes on them in lectures. This requires them to be well-organized. We also have an online drug assessment 'authentic world'. We even have an online 'virtual family and community', which we use as a learning tool. Students do need to be computer savvy nowadays or they are disadvantaged. 99

- Blackboard and web-CT are web-based VLEs, which are interactive and easily accessed on and off campus, once you have your login details.
- Moodle is an alternative to the above.
- Wikis are community blogs designed to be added to by anyone who has access to them. Many universities create their own for nursing students.
- A weblog is a personal journal or diary intended for public viewing. Some universities use blogs to get students to reflect (see Chapter 12) on their experiences. Remember confidentiality, anyone can access a weblog (NMC 2008).
- Podcasting is sharing sound files and sometimes powerpoint slides. These can be accessed on a computer or MP3/MP4 player having been posted on a website by a lecturer. This is not intended to replace attending lectures, but to enhance your learning and are useful for revision. Vodcasts are podcasts that are video.

5.5 **Referencing**

Student comment

" Be clear about the use of references, they are essential for every piece of work as they show reasoning behind why nurses do what they do. Understand how to use them and find out exactly how the university wants them presented. "

Your written assignments at university will need to make reference to the literature. But what does this mean and why does it matter? The following explains.

Referencing is what you are doing when you indicate to the reader of your assignment what books and journals or websites etc. (references) you have used to support your work. You make links in the body of your writing to the list of references, which you will place at the end of your work. This is important as all statements, opinions and conclusions that you have read in articles or books or on websites *must* be acknowledged. You may directly quote, paraphrase (put in to your own words) or summarize. Student nurses *must* use references in their written work to support their argument and to show their understanding of the theory and how it relates to practice.

? **Stop and think** Theory/practice links explained

When you recall the first-year bioscience lecture on bones, muscles and joints, you realize you understand more about the needs of an 85-year-old with a fractured neck or femur. When you read further about the prognosis in such a case, it highlights the importance of rehabilitation and mobilization of older people with such conditions.

As the module assignment was a care study, you decided to focus on this patient's rehabilitation and mobilization after surgery. In it you draw together (i.e. link) your *knowledge from the lecture*, from *your reading* and from your *experience working with the patient*. You write about how care was planned and implemented in practice, and make reference to the additional reading you have done.

If you do all this, you are making good theory/practice links. Remember the phrase: theory without practise is empty, practise without theory is blind.

So which referencing system is required?

Student comment

66 Grow to love your referencing guidelines and follow them to the letter. You don't have to learn them off by heart in the first week, it will come to you. Don't re-invent the wheel. 99

There are many different ways to reference but the two main methods in use are Harvard and Vancouver.

* The Harvard system uses the author's name and year of publication within the text of the work and the reference list at the end is alphabetical by first author's surname.
* The Vancouver system numbers each entry within the text as it occurs. So, if Hart (2010) was the 6th book you referred to in your essay, then the full reference would appear as number 6 in the reference list.

! Fact box Examples of reference lists

Harvard

Davies C, Finlay L and Bullman A (2000) *Changing practice in health and social care.* Sage/Open University, London.

Mason J (2002) *Qualitative researching* (2nd edn). Sage Publications, London.

Nursing and Midwifery Council (NMC) (2008) *The code: standards of conduct, performance and ethics for nurses and midwives.* Nursing and Midwifery Council, London.

Quinn FM and Hughes S (2007) *Quinn's principles and practice of nurse education* (2nd edn). Nelson Thornes, Cheltenham.

Vancouver

Price D. Freedom from restraint. In: Brown C, Frank P (eds) *Managing psychiatric care.* London: Johnson, 2000.

Rockingham E. *Study skills for mentors.* Exeter: Jackson, 2011.

Your university is likely to require a certain style of referencing and it is most likely that this will be *based* on either Harvard or Vancouver. However, the particular details required, the order they appear in the reference list and the formatting will vary from one university to another. It is essential, therefore, that you obtain a copy of your university department's reference guidelines and follow this *carefully* and *consistently*.

Why and how to reference

Student comment

66 I always prefer to not use direct quotes and find paraphrasing best, it makes referencing easier. 99

Academic work demands that you read widely to show your understanding. To use another person's work *without acknowledgement* is considered to be plagiarism (see Fact box) and is serious academic misconduct. When referencing you put into your text the origin of any ideas that you use. Sometimes you will read texts that support your own view (e.g. the importance of people with learning disability leading ordinary lives in the community, and having families of their own). You may also disagree with what you read (e.g. the writing of those that believe people with learning disability should live in village communities away from mainstream society). To show you have read and thought about both sides of the argument is excellent.

The actual 'reference' itself is a recognized shorthand means of describing a document, or part of a document, with enough details such as author(s) and title to enable others to identify and locate it.

References may be categorized as coming from *primary* or *secondary* sources. A primary reference indicates that you have used original material. If you have read the text 'Cultural awareness in nursing and health care' by Karen Holland and Christine Hogg, this would be a primary source, e.g.

Holland K and Hogg C (2001) *Cultural awareness in nursing and health care.* Arnold, London.

If you have *not* read their book, but have read *about* their work in a book by another author, this would be a secondary source. It is preferable to use primary sources as it is wise not to rely on the interpretation of another author. However, if you cannot find the primary source, then you may use secondary referencing. In so doing, you must show in the text that it is work cited by another.

When referencing you should refer to the author whose work you *have* read, telling the reader that he or she cites another source, which you name. You must indicate

> **! Fact box** Plagiarism and academic misconduct
>
> Plagiarism means to present another person's work as if it is your own. This could be the work of a class mate or a published author. Plagiarism is academic misconduct. If you are found guilty of plagiarism you may be asked to leave the programme. Do note that most universities have plagiarism-detection tools. Also, nurse teachers are familiar with the core texts that students use.

> **! Fact box**
>
> Some universities may require you to list your secondary sources as well as the primary sources. You must read your own uni guidelines carefully.

the page number of the source, as shown in the examples below. This can be done in several ways:

Mason (2002: 92) cites the work of Coffey (1999) who proposed. . .

Coffey (1999, cited in Mason 2002: 92) proposed. . .

or:

Mason (2002: 92, citing Coffey 1999) argues. . .

There are variants but these alternatives will do for most situations. The author that should be in the reference list should be Mason (2002) not Coffey (1999).

Citing references in the text

In the Harvard system, cited publications are referred to in the text by giving the author's surname and the year of publication in one of the forms shown below.

If the author's name occurs naturally in the sentence, the year is given in parentheses (brackets), e.g.

In a recent study Alexander (2004) argued that…

If, however, the name does not occur naturally in the sentence, both name and year are given in parentheses:

A recent study (Alexander 2004) suggests that…

If there are two authors, the surnames of both should be given:

Matthews and Jones (2001) have proposed that…

If there are more than two authors the surname of the first author only should be given, followed by *et al.* in italics:

Wilson *et al.* (2000) conclude that…

However, *all* the contributors must be listed in the reference list.

Reference lists

Every reference that has been used in the text must be listed at the end of your work, in a particular order that allows the reader to locate them quickly and easily. In the Harvard system, authors are listed alphabetically and then chronologically, as follows:

- Single-author works are listed alphabetically by authors' surnames but if an author has more than one work cited, then these are listed chronologically (earliest first, e.g. 2001, 2007). If the same author has more than one work cited for the same year, then avoid ambiguity by using 'a', 'b', etc. (e.g. 2008a, 2008b).

> Nursing and Midwifery Council (NMC) (2008a) *The code: standards of conduct, performance and ethics for nurses and midwives.* Nursing and Midwifery Council, London.

> Nursing and Midwifery Council (NMC) (2008b) *Standards to support learning and assessment in practice* (2nd edn). Nursing and Midwifery Council, London.

- Two-author works are listed alphabetically by first author's name and then by second author's name, e.g.

  > Jones F (2008)

  > Jones F and Smith B (2008)

  > Jones F and Taylor G (2000)

- Multi-author works are listed alphabetically by first author's surname then chrono-logically, e.g.

  > Jones F (2008)

  > Jones F and Smith B (2008)

  > Jones F and Taylor G (2000)

  > Jones F, Smith B and Brown M (2000)

  > Jones F, Brown M and Taylor G (2002)

This is because in the text you would have cited Jones *et al.* and so the reader would not know who the other authors were; instead they can locate the reference easily by looking up Jones as first author followed by year.

! **Fact box** Internet sources also must be listed

In addition to the usual information, you will need to make a note of the URL (website) and state on what date you accessed the information.

Exercise 5.3

Imagine you have used for your assignment the book called *Learning disability: toward inclusion* edited by Bob Gates and published by Elsevier in Edinburgh in 2007. You have used Chapter 15, pages 281–300 by Sue Hart called 'Health and health promotion'. (See reference list on page 195 for the answer.) How would you reference this using the Harvard system?

Summary

Teaching and learning in a university is quite different from what it was at school or college. You will increase your chances of success by making the most of the opportunities open to you and engaging in the spirit of adult education. For those who need to be reminded; lecturers do not chase adult learners to submit work; it is down to you to do what is asked, when it is asked. Your success, or otherwise is in your hands. The best learning in class-rooms comes when all students engage in the activity, be it role-play or EBL. Enjoy the variety of learning that a university education offers. Learning well, positions you to tackle your assessments, as the next chapter shows.

■ Top tips

- Thinking of yourself as *working in partnership* with your lecturers and others to fulfil your goals is helpful.
- Understanding your own role in learning is a key to your success.
- Be an active learner; engage, be inquisitive.
- Read widely: books, journal articles, and health related topics in a quality newspaper. It will broaden your knowledge base and help your written work.
- Don't waste time writing up neat notes after a lecture, perfect your note-taking and use the time you save reading.
- Teachers *always* want to see more in your assignment than their regurgitated lecture notes.
- All statements, opinions, conclusions and so on, taken from another writer's work, should be acknowledged.
- However you reference, *you must be consistent*.
- Always follow your own uni guidelines.

■ Online resource centre

You can find further advice to help you get the most from your time at university by going online to **www.oxfordtextbooks.co.uk/orc/hart/** where you can find links to websites on learning styles, academic levels and tips on accessing electronic resources and finding materials using search tools.

■ References

Atherton JS (2005) *Bloom's taxonomy learning and teaching*. Available: http://www.learningandteaching.info/learning/bloomtax.htm.

Bloom BS (1956) *Taxonomy of educational objectives*. Published by Allyn and Bacon, Boston, MA. Copyright (c) 1984 by Pearson Education

Honey P and Mumford A (1992) *The manual of learning styles*. Peter Honey, Maidenhead.

Knowles M (1984) *The adult learner: a neglected species* (3rd edn). Gulf Publishing, Houston, TX.

University of Surrey (n.d.) *Academic levels*. Available: http://portal.surrey.ac.uk/pls/portal/docs/PAGE/REGISTRY/MOD/ABOUTLEV.DOC

■ Websites

L2L Enquiry-based learning: http://www.som.surrey.ac.uk/learningtolearn/intro.asp?section=2

Smith MK (2002) 'Malcolm Knowles, informal adult education, self-direction and anadragogy', *The Encyclopaedia of Informal Education*: http://www.infed.org/thinkers/et-knowl.htm

Study skills guide to successful assessments

Liz Rockingham

The aims of this chapter are:

➤ To outline self-help activities to aid your learning

➤ To introduce you to some assessment methods

➤ To give guidance how to undertake these

➤ To direct you to online resources to support your study skills development

As a university student you learn *actively* as you participate in and contribute to your own learning. This chapter will help you to develop the basic *learning* and *academic skills* you will need in order to be successful in this. As you read you may note that many of the skills discussed will be useful in your *placements* as well. Chapter 5 introduced some of the teaching and learning techniques lecturers use, but adult learning is a two-way process. The following is central to your success.

6.1 Student learning activities

Reading

Reading is a primary route to effective learning. Knowing what to read, how to read and how to access the required literature are important skills. Reading may include journal articles, case histories, library books or recommended texts you may have bought (such as this). Developing good reading habits will serve you well. It is one of the best ways to consolidate your understanding and make theory/practice links. But what is good reading?

Reading actively means engaging with what you read, and may require you to re-read certain passages and take notes. Skim reading or scanning the pages first helps you to 'tune in' and also helps you to be selective and ensure the reading is right for you (i.e. that it addresses the question that you have). Learning speed-reading techniques may be helpful (see online resource).

Student comment

❝ When you have read something, see if you can write a list of the main points without looking at it. Then check to see if your points reflect accurately what you have read. ❞

Literature searching

You will be advised at uni how to search for information online, e.g. using databases and in the library. You will be given an Athens password to access these databases. See the online resource for more information.

Note-taking

Student comment

❝ Make sure that you go back over your lecture notes, especially when you had difficulty understanding. You will be glad you did when it all falls into place! ❞

Taking notes involves summarizing what is being said in the lecture to read later in order to remember what was said. Notes should prompt your recollection of the topic. They are not intended to be a word-for-word account of the lecture. They are not a substitute for the additional reading your lecturer has recommended.

Student reflection on poor note-taking

See Figure 6.1.

'In these notes I wrote anywhere on the page and seemed to think using colours would help. There is no structure. I don't remember this lecture. I was too busy trying to write everything, that I didn't soak any of it in'.

Student reflection on better note-taking

See Figure 6.2.

'This is more recent note-taking. It is not as colourful but it is much more organized. I have learnt that I do not need to write down everything. I can revise from these notes logically'.

*Research Bolam test! <u>Dec 2007</u>

Consent

Consent is when a voluntary decision is made by a sufficiently competent or autonomous person on the basis of adequate information.

'Patients on their journey through the healthcare system are entitled to be treated with respect and honesty and to be included wherever possible in decisions about their care.'

* Consent forms must be used wherever possible*

* All hospitals should be PALS.

```
P  A  L  S
A  D  I  E
T  V  A  R
I  I  I  V
E  S  S  I
N  O  O  C
T  R  N  E
   Y
```

* Gillick competence

<u>Implied consent</u>
Where we do not require a signature,e.g. blood pressure.

<u>Clinical side</u>
Where clients have an ethical right to make their own decisions.

<u>Legal side</u>
Consent must be obtained or client can file for assault.

* Consent can ensure mental and physical improvement

Figure 6.1 Example of poor note-taking in a lecture on consent

Student comment

66 As boring and sad as it may sound, get a study group going! You may not understand something, but maybe a fellow student can help break the information down. You're all in the same situation with the same goal, so help each other! 99

Research 1

Evidence-based practice

Learning to do nursing care with good reason or scientific based

Need to consider:

Scientific enquiry—audits, statistics, etc
Effective knowledge management
Effective change systems
Incentives!

How to achieve:

- Ask the right questions
- Find best evidence
- Being critical
- Acting on the evidence
- Appraise your performance

P = Patient, problem
I = Intervention
C = Comparison
O = Outcome

Finding the best evidence
Searching the best evidence
CINAHL, MEDLINE—primary sources
Secondary sources
Systematic reviews
Meta-analysis

Research Paradigms	Positive Paradigm	Positive Paradigm
Validity	What is it meant to measure?	Is there full access?
Reliability	Does the research change?	Is it different in other areas?
Generalizability	Is it available to all sources?	Do all theories apply?

Figure 6.2 **Example of good note-taking in a research lecture**

Class tests and examinations

Student comment

❝Don't leave revising until the last minute; it doesn't do you any favours. It's amazing what you can learn and remember in just an hour or two of an evening.❞

Tests and exams are useful for you to gauge your progress and direct the focus of your future studying. They also help teachers to support you as needed, as well as assessing you. Test fear can re-stimulate some childhood anxieties, which many adults struggle to overcome. It helps to see tests as an aid to your learning, rather than making judgements about you.

Nurse teacher comment

❝In practice, as well as in lectures, you will learn a lot by observing, listening and participating. The more engaged you are in your learning, the more you will absorb and the more successful you will be. ❞

6.2 **How you will be assessed**

This part of the chapter will help you to understand some of the different methods of assessment and give you ideas for approaching each one. It will explain what the assessment guidelines are asking for. This chapter will explain how to plan and structure an assignment, but it will not focus in-depth on academic writing styles, instead please access the help available with this skill at the online resource centre).

! Fact box

All universities have their own guidelines for how to present written work. It is essential that you know what your university requires of you. The examples in this chapter are for illustration only.

· · · A word about Objectivity and subjectivity

To be objective is to be impartial, neutral and present facts in an argument in a logical detached way. Think of a judge summing up a case in court and, based on the evidence, making a judgement. Your academic work is more convincing if you refer to the work of other people to back up the point you want to make. In an essay this is done through reference to the literature (books, journals). In a discussion this is done by using the name of the person whose work you have read. For example, in a discussion about 'expert patients' to add 'as long ago as 1951 Carl Rogers wrote about the notion of the "client as the expert"' would be to give some history and credibility to this way of thinking.

To be subjective is to base your ideas and opinions on your own feelings and emotions. What you think and feel is of value, and you will have opportunities during the course to share your own perspective on issues, e.g. through reflection (see Chapter 12). However, if in a discussion you present your own considered view, when you have also demonstrated you have thought about the views of others (through listening, reading and research), your *informed* opinion will be more valued by others.

> **! Fact box** Examples of methods of assessments used on pre registration nursing programmes
>
> Essays give you an opportunity to link experience in practice to the theory that you have been taught in class, literature searched and read about yourself. In your essay you demonstrate your understanding by supporting your work with references.
>
> Care studies are where you write about a patient or group of patients you have cared for. When doing this you make links to the theory you have learned and your reading, with reference to the care given.
>
> Reading logs require you to discuss a book or article that you have read and consider how it has informed you and your practice
>
> Literature reviews require you to search for, and then read and summarize, a range of articles and/or books on a topic (see 6.8 below).
>
> Examinations can be 'seen' or 'open book' where you are told the questions in advance, or unseen. Exams require you to demonstrate your knowledge of the subject (e.g. nursing care of a cardiac patient), the underpinning theory (e.g. biological science) and the application to practice. Sometimes exams have multiple-choice questions (MCQs, see 6.9 below).
>
> Online examinations, e.g. bio science or drug calculations and pharmacology, using Software such as 'Authentic world'.

Exactly how your programme is assessed will have been planned when the course was developed. The assessments you must do will be determined by your university and the requirements of the NMC. For example, a regulation at your university may be that every student must sit at least one unseen examination per year (or per level). However, wherever you are studying, it is likely that there will be a range of ways that your knowledge and understanding will be assessed.

6.3 **Some things to consider before starting working on your assessments**

Student comment

66 Don't leave assignments until the night before, but also don't start them too early, like months ahead. Starting too early can result in too much time/energy expenditure; you keep changing and rewriting your essay. 99

Later, this chapter looks at each of these methods of assessment in more detail and gives advice about how to approach each one. We have done this as they all have different requirements. However, for all assessments you must consider the following checklist for submitting course work:

- What is the date for submission?
- How long have you got to complete the work?
- Do you understand the guidelines?
- Is there any reason that may prevent you from submitting on time?
- At what level is your assessment going to be marked?
- How should the work be presented?
- What referencing system is required?
- How to submit (how, where and number of copies)

What is the date for submission?

If you are unsure why this is important, go back to Chapter 4. Plan your work mindful of all your other commitments. You need to be writing assessments whilst in placement.

How long have you got to complete the work?

See Chapter 4 for advice about prioritizing your work.

Do you understand the guidelines?

For each assessment you will receive guidelines such as in the example below. How detailed this is and what it says will be determined by your teachers. At a minimum you will have a title, submission date and word count. The example gives students a number of guidelines. Note there is no exact title here, rather a guide to write about one of three areas.

Example assessment guidelines

Essential Nursing Skills, level 4, 20 credits

An essay to focus on professional values, communication or patient/client assessment

Length: 1200 words

Submission date: 28 November 2010

Presentation:

- Your work must be word processed and one side only.
- It must be double-line spaced.
- The pages must be numbered.

- It must be within the word limit (+ or − 10%).
- It must include a reference list.
- It must be submitted in a clear fronted plastic folder.
- Do not put each sheet into a plastic sleeve.
- Do not staple the pages together.
- Make sure you name is on your submission (normally there will be a sheet available for you to fill in and submit with your assignment).
- If you use examples from practice they *must* be anonymous and respect confidentiality.

Structure:

- Your essay should have an introduction, a main body and conclusion.
- Sub-headings are not needed. Use paragraphs to give direction to the work.

Content:

The essay question is broad to allow you to select the topic of your choice. There is no right or wrong answer.

Introduction:

Indicate here how you are going to approach the essay. Include:

- A statement identifying your future field of practice.
- A statement indicating which of the three areas you will write about.

Main body:
To include:

- A brief description of the topic you have chosen (e.g. the professional value of confidentiality).
- Refer back to what you were taught in the module and show how your learning and additional reading has influenced your practice.

Conclusion:

- Briefly summarize what you have said.
- Include ideas for how you can develop your role in the future.
- Do not include new material.

Referencing:

- Literature should be correctly referenced using the Harvard System.
- There is no minimum or maximum number of references.
- Notes from lectures cannot be used as a reference.

Is there any reason that may prevent you from submitting on time?

Under certain circumstances it may be possible to obtain an extension to the submission date, allowing more time to complete the work. The giving of extensions is monitored; they are not given automatically. Supporting evidence, e.g. a letter confirming you have been called for jury service, may be needed. You may be refused an extension if it is thought your circumstances do not justify extra time. If you need an extension, apply well in advance of the submission date. Apply if your need is genuine, but remember, extra time gained by an extension for one assessment is lost on your next assessment.

> **! Fact box** Who gives extensions?
>
> It is usual practice to have named lecturers to give extensions. These individuals talk to each other and keep records of who has been given an extension and who has been turned down. So if your request has been turned down, it will not be agreed by another lecturer; so save yourself the embarrassment of asking around. Accept the decision and work hard to submit a good attempt on time.

> **... A word about** Personal mitigating circumstances (PMC)
>
> All universities take into consideration genuine and verifiable extenuating or mitigating circumstances, which may have prevented a student attending an examination or submitting course work by the deadline, or which may have affected their performance in that assessment. Evidence will be required. Make sure you let someone know if you experience problems such as:
>
> • Bereavement involving a close relative or a friend (evidence: death certificate copy).
> • Accident or illness requiring hospitalization (hospital letter, sick note).
> • Infectious disease (hospital letter, sick note).
> • Burglary/theft (police crime report).

At what level is your assessment going to be marked?

As we said in Chapter 5, all the assessed work you do will be marked according to grading criteria. These exist to ensure fairness. Be familiar with the grading criteria *before you start writing*.

The example grading criteria at the online resource gives an idea of the requirements for a level 4 assessment. Note the main areas being assessed and the spread of marks:

- Knowledge and understanding 40%.
- Cognitive skills 30%.
- Presentation and referencing 20%.
- Integration of theory and practice 10%.

Your work must pay attention to all these areas. To do well in 'knowledge and understanding' you must show the marker what you know about the subject. To demonstrate your cognitive skills you must show you are thinking about this information, e.g. how are you making links from this to other things you have been taught?

Note 40% of the marks are available for 'knowledge and understanding' and only 10% for 'integration of theory and practice'. At level 4 you are not yet expected to be able to integrate theory and practice to a high level. This more complex skill will be acquired later (remember Bloom in Chapter 5).

Thinking about the available marks is helpful to guide your level of effort. If you present and reference your work as instructed, you can expect to a lot of the 20% available marks; but however expertly you do this, you can only get 20%, no more. It makes sense to pay the necessary level of attention to all four areas.

The language used in assessments also indicates the level you need to work at, e.g. describe or discuss will be used at level 4. Later your assessments will contain words such as criticize, analyse and evaluate, as these are higher level activities. See the online resource for more details about language used in assessments.

+ ....

Exercise 6.1

Study the example grading criteria at the online resource or the one in use at your university. Use this information to focus your work.

....

How should the work be presented?

To be successful you need to know precisely how the module or unit leader is asking you to present your work, and then do as you are asked. Even if you cannot understand why a request is made, still do it. For example, you may be asked 'not to put each sheet of your essay in a plastic sleeve'. In this case it is because of the time needed to remove pages from sleeves in order to mark them.

What referencing system is required?

See your university guidelines and Chapter 5 for more advice.

How to submit (how, where and number of copies)

See your university guidelines for this and, again, do exactly as you are asked, in good time.

This chapter will now guide you to start thinking about your assessments.

6.4 **Essays**

Imagine you have the following level 4, 1200 word essay to write:

'Effective communication is an important part of a nurse's role. With reference to your recent practice, outline some of the barriers to effective communication and give some examples of good practice that you have seen.'

First, take some thinking and planning time; this is an important first step in the process. Essay writing is best tackled in stages. Start by:

- Re-reading the title several times to determine exactly what is required.
- Read through all the guidelines you are given.
- Underline key words and phrases, checking understanding with a dictionary, if necessary.

<u>Effective communication</u> is an important part of a <u>nurse's role</u>. With reference to <u>your recent practice,</u> outline some of the <u>barriers</u> to effective communication and give some <u>examples of good practice</u> that you have seen.

?   Stop and think

What do you think the focus of this assignment is?

Answer: linking what you have seen in practice with the reading you have done about 'communication', and writing about the obstacles to this and the effective methods you have observed.

Student comment

66 *If you do not understand a word in an assignment question always look up the definition. Don't attempt to guess what it means, as if it is wrong you could fail your assessment.* 99

Nurse teacher comment

66 If you do not understand what you are being asked to do, seek help from an academic tutor. 99

Planning the essay

Plan how you are going to proceed on one side of A4. Start by thinking about what effective communication means to you and about barriers (obstructions) to this that you may have seen in practice. Ask yourself, is the question asking about effective communication between patients and nurses, or between professionals? As it does not say exactly, it is up to you to decide how you are going to approach the answer and signal this to the reader in your introduction. As it is part of a nurse's role to communicate with patients, their families and fellow professionals, you could include some examples from all these three areas. To answer this way is not 'right' or 'wrong', it is simply the decision made in this case about how to approach the question.

Student comment

66 Do not change your assignment if you feel you are answering the question, just because a friend says they are taking a different direction to you. As long as the question is being answered, you should be OK, and who's to say your friend is right! 99

Although the essay asks you to refer to what you may have seen in practice, you must support this with reference to literature. So next:

- Consider what sources of information will help you answer the question (e.g. module set books, journal articles). Allow enough searching time to find these sources and then read, making notes, and marking useful passages on post it notes. Noting page numbers and references as you read (author, date, title, publisher, etc.) will save time later when typing your reference list.

- From what you have read, decide what you want to include in your essay. Jot down ideas for answering each aspect of the question. It helps at this stage to think in themes. What is effective communication? What are some of the barriers to it?

Note useful examples, definitions, quotations and references, as well as possible points of argument. Remember, in deciding what to include and what to discard, the key word is *relevance* to the title.

Writing the essay

Usually this requires writing a first draft, editing this and making alterations, cutting and pasting, as necessary, then writing a final copy. If time is short, it is possible to write up a neat copy from a thorough plan.

At this stage it is important to concentrate on expressing your ideas clearly and developing a flow for your argument, so that the marker can follow your thinking.

Introduction

Show how you intend to answer the question. If you plan to draw on your placement experience in a mental health outreach team, say so here.

The main body of the essay

This is where you answer the question. You may have chosen to do this by:

- exploring the meaning of 'effective communication' (e.g. open body language, speaking clearly, checking understanding); then

- highlighting three examples from practice where you witnessed barriers to effective communication (e.g. no hearing-aid inserted, background noise or speaking too quickly for the person) plus three examples of good practice (using pictures to aid communication with someone with learning disability or who is unable to speak, avoiding the use of jargon, re-wording an explanation a person did not understand).

Consider how what you have read relates to your experience in practice. Include 'signpost' phrases to show the marker where the argument is leading. For example: 'Having looked at the strengths of ...'; 'Possible criticisms of it are ...'; 'Conversely ...'. It is also useful to relate the points you make back to the question to bring out their relevance. For example, 'another barrier to effective communication in practice was ...'

Conclusion

Here you draw your argument together. The conclusion must follow logically from the preceding argument. Do not include new material. If something is important enough to be discussed in your essay it needs to be in the main body.

When writing, try to use simple and direct language. Be careful to distinguish between your own ideas and those of other authors. Acknowledge quotes '...' and give references. Remember to keep to the word limit (usually within a 10% margin either way) or you will be penalized (Giminez 2007).

Advice on editing (proof-reading) your first draft

Always read through your essay carefully, with a critical eye, to be sure what you have written does what you need it to. Check for the following:

- Relevance: does the essay really answer the question set? Has anything important been omitted? Can anything be removed because it is repetitive, unnecessary and not contributing to the answer?

- Structure: is there a logical order? Is it well organized? Is there development and unfolding of your argument throughout? Is the argument 'sign-posted'?

- Clarity of expression: is it clearly written? Would rephrasing or expanding any points make them clearer? Would an example be helpful? Are the tenses correct? Check spelling, punctuation, and sentence and paragraph construction. The spell and grammar checker on your computer is helpful. Reading your essay aloud can help to check grammar. Does it sound correct and make sense? If not, use different words to explain the point another way. Does it sound clearer now? If so, re-write your sentence based on what you just said. The more you practice, the easier it gets.

- Accuracy: is all the evidence used cited correctly in the text? Is your reference list correct? Have you followed the guidelines for presentation? Is the word number within the range?

Final draft

Make all the necessary adjustments after the proof-reading. Keep your focus. It is not unusual at this stage to be impatient, to want to get it finished and submitted; but your success depends on you getting this right. However 'fed up' you may feel with the essay at this point, it is not as bad as you will feel if you fail, and especially if it was for something you could easily have rectified earlier.

Preparing to submit

Student comment

❝ Have a list of how work needs to be presented so that when finishing something you can just go through it and check that it's double-spaced, correct font size and so on. ❞

Print your work as instructed and check before submission if all the pages have been printed. Also are they in the right order? If there was more than one title, is it obvious which essay you selected? Teachers will not guess. Make sure you attach any necessary information, such as a top sheet. Fill this out correctly.

Nurse teacher comment

❝ You should think of all the things that could go wrong and then double-check they do not. Even down to the actual submission, things can go haywire. A new student knew she had to put her essay in a box, but unfortunately got muddled about where she should go to do this and ended up in an office submitting her essay into a shredder. True story! ❞

The above are not hard and fast rules; they are suggestions to help support you when writing your first essay. Thinking is a very important part of essay writing. Allow time for this.

6.5 **Numeracy**

Competency in basic mathematics is essential for safe nursing practice. Nurses must be confident in their own skills to calculate, e.g:

- The correct amount of a drug to administer to the adult or child.
- A patient's fluid balance.
- The nutritional needs for a person.
- The weight of a patient and their body mass index.
- The intravenous fluid required and the rate that it should be administered.

Many people have difficulties with numeracy (numbers) and if you are concerned, seek the support you need as early as possible. You may not have 'liked' this subject at school, but this may be because it was not taught well. For this reason you may have (ungrounded) fears that you cannot master it; but you can and help is available. Get the help you need and there is every chance you will succeed; but bury your head in the sand, and you risk failure.

Nurse teacher comment

❝ The NMC require that first-year student's ability with numbers is assessed. So the more you practice, the better you will do. It builds confidence. ❞

Numeracy: what exactly do you need to know?

The good news is that you do not need to understand algebra or geometry. You do need to know:

- The relationship between kilogram (kg), gram (g), milligram (mg) and microgram (mcg), i.e. that there are 1000 g in 1 kg.
- The relationship between litre (l) and millilitre (ml), i.e. that there are 1000 ml in 1 l.

Also you need to be able to:

- add;
- subtract (take away);
- divide;
- multiply;
- work with decimals and fractions.

Common weights and volumes used in drug calculations are:

- 1 kg (kilogram) = 1000 g (gram);
- 1 g = 1000 mg (milligram);
- 1 mg = 1000 microgram (microgram are always written in full on prescriptions to avoid misinterpretation);
- 1 l (litre) = 1000 ml (millilitre).

To change from a large unit to a smaller unit multiply, e.g. gram to milligram needs to x 1000.

To change from a smaller unit to a larger unit divide by 1000, e.g. gram to kilogram.

Another way of doing this is to move the decimal point, e.g. to change 0.4 g to mg you multiply by 1000, but as there are three zeros in 1000, you could also move the decimal point three places to the right.

Normally the decimal point after the 400 is not shown, but is not wrong if you do show it.

Stock volume means the quality of drug in a given amount, e.g. there may be 125 mg of a drug in 5 ml of liquid.

$$\curvearrowright\curvearrowright\curvearrowright$$
$$0.400$$
$$400.00$$

Figure 6.3 To change 0.4 g to mg you will multiply by 1000. But as there are three zeros in 1000 you can move the decimal point three places to the right. The arrow shows the movement of the decimal point three places to the right

+..

Exercise 6.2 Numeracy

Try the following eight questions (answers can be found at the end of the chapter)

Key: X = multiply; / or ÷ = divide

1. 32 x 4 =

2. 1239 + 3178 =

3. 28 x 0.5 =

4. 40/10 =

5. 0.3 x 9 =

6. Convert 2300 mg into g =

7. Which is bigger 40 ml or 0.3 l =

8. There are 4 patients in a bay aged 60, 85, 72 and 63. What is the mean (average) age?

....

Drug calculations

There are several ways of working out drug dosages. A popular method is seen in Figure 6.4.

Now try the four questions below, but first make sure you have what you need (e.g. calculator, pen and paper). You might find it helpful to have the formula written down as well.

1. A person in your care has been prescribed 1 gm of paracetamol. The tablets you have are 500 mg each. How many tablets would you give them?

2. A child has been prescribed 62.5 mg of phenoximethylpenicillin. The label on the bottle states there are 125 mg in 5 ml. How many ml do you give her?

3. A person who has epilepsy has been prescribed sodium valporate 300 mg. The available stock is 200 mg in 5 ml. How much does the person need?

$$\frac{\text{What you want (dose)}}{\text{What you have got (stock)}} \times \text{Stock value}$$

Example:

240 mg calpol prescribed for a child

Stock volume = 120 mg in 5 ml

$$\frac{240}{120} \times 5 = 2 \times 5 = 10$$

Therefore need 10 ml.

Figure 6.4 How to work out a drug dosage

4. A person with learning disability in a community service has a dental abscess. The dentist has prescribed Metronidazole 400 mg. The local chemist has dispensed 200 mg tablets. Use your preferred method to work this out.

If you found these difficult, why not try some of the online resources that are suggested. We have known many students who are terrified of maths at the beginning of the course but with work, become proficient, so that they can do all the calculations that are required of them.

Nurse teacher comment

66 Do not be surprised to find that different resources explain calculations using a variety of methods. What is important is to double-check you have got it right. Find the method that works for you and stick to it. 99

6.6 **Care study**

Imagine you have been given the following title:

'Identify a person you nursed on your last placement and discuss the plan of care that was implemented for them. Focus on a person who has a physical, learning or communication difficulty to illustrate how your care was individualized.'

Again, start by unpicking the question, noting any key words and phrases.

'Identify a patient or client you nursed during a recent placement. Discuss the plan of care that was implemented for them during their admission. Focus on a person who has a physical, learning or communication difficulty and show how your care was individualized.'

Questions to ask yourself

- What is the focus of the module that this case study is the assessment for? If it is a health and social care module, you may wish to show your knowledge about both these areas.

- What skills, knowledge and attitudes do I need to show to achieve the module outcomes?

- What is the relevance of this work to my development as a nurse?

Thinking time

Thinking about the question is an essential starting point. You are being asked to write about one person, not a group. Think about what you need to say. Why am I being asked this question?

Who shall I choose to base my care study on?

Imagine you have nursed each individual below, in the last 3 months:

- Sam, who has Down's Syndrome, in hospital with a chest infection.
- John, a 73-year-old man, on a medical ward, following a recent cerebral-vascular accident (stroke).
- Lily is 2 years old and has asthma.

All the people above could be subjects in this care plan, but:

- Why choose them in particular?
- What model of care was used in their care and could this be a helpful framework for the care plan?

There are many models of nursing. These guide the type of assessment, planning, implementation and evaluation necessary for the holistic care for each individual. When planning care for a patient, their individual needs and wishes must be taken into account to ensure that their care is individualized (i.e. right for them) and holistic (that is paying the necessary attention to their particular physical, psychological and social needs, etc.). Whilst on placement you may have worked in an area that has its own model to suit the needs of the patients that are cared for in that setting.

How to structure the answer?

Start by introducing the person on whom you will base your answer. Identify their nursing need (i.e. physical, learning or communication difficulty) and the care-planning tool you will write about (Barrett et al. 2009). Imagine you have selected 'John' above. Following the cerebral-vascular accident, he has physical and communication difficulties. His care plan will need to suit his individual needs. As the focus of the module assessment is on individualized and holistic nursing care, consider the skills, knowledge and attitudes you need to be able to demonstrate to achieve the module outcomes. As this is a level-4 assessment, at the minimum you must show knowledge and understanding of individualized and holistic, nursing care planning.

For the main body, use elements from the care model as a framework for your care plan (an example of a care planning tool by Roper, Logan and Tierney appears below). You

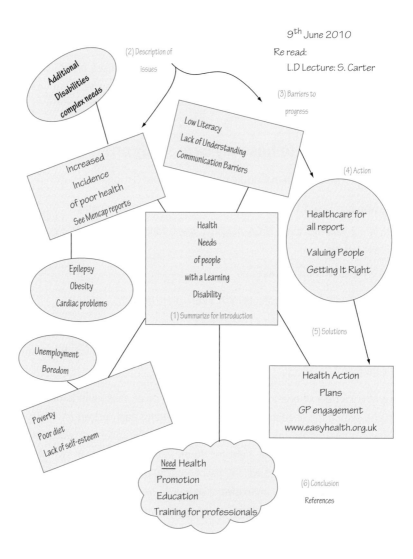

Figure 6.5 Spider diagram

will also need to read more about John's specific conditions and the effect this will have on his care. Think about using a technique such as a 'mind map' (Buzan 1993) or 'spider diagram' (see Figure 6.5) when formulating your answer. Let your ideas flow freely and then tighten them up later.

Now, for example, write about John's needs using the headings in Roper, Logan and Tierney's model as follows. Use supporting literature as references to demonstrate your knowledge.

- Maintaining a safe environment:
  - John not aware of his left side of his body.
  - Difficulty standing; encourage him to call for help when he wishes to stand or walk.

- Communication:
  - John has dysphasia, encourage him to speak, ensure communication boards are available to avoid frustration.
- Breathing:
  - Ensure John has a patent airway.
  - John has difficulty swallowing, so needs thickened fluids to avoid aspiration.
- Eating and drinking:
  - Ensure John has sufficient thickened fluid, use a fluid chart.
  - Refer to dietician.
  - Use a food chart to ensure adequate nutrition.
- Elimination:
  - Ensure urine bottle is where John can see it.
  - John is prone to constipation, encourage high-fibre foods and monitor output.
- Washing and dressing:
  - Assist John with hygiene needs.
  - Encourage John to help himself.
- Controlling temperature:
  - Aim for John to be apyrexial (i.e. to have a normal temperature).
  - Take temperature daily.
- Mobilization:
  - Encourage him to walk down the ward using a tripod.
  - John is unaware of his left side, encourage him to focus more on it.
  - Help John to do exercises the physiotherapist recommends.
  - Encourage John's family to participate.
- Working and playing:
  - John enjoys listening to Radio 4.
- Expressing sexuality:
  - John gets embarrassed when being cared for by younger female nurses.
  - Ensure privacy and dignity.
- Sleeping:
  - John has difficulty sleeping unless he has two pillows under his head and one under his left arm.
- Death and dying:
  - He does not wish to be resuscitated and has discussed this with his family.

Conclusion

Here you summarize the evidence used to show how the care of John was individualized. You could also note a couple of points where you believed the care was not so good and make recommendations (suggestions) about how care could be improved in the future. Likewise, you could note if care was excellent and say why this was the case.

How will I know it is good enough to submit?

Proof-read your work, asking yourself, have I answered the question? Have I met the module outcomes? If not, add new material, eliminate repetition or anything that does not answer the question. Be ruthless. If you can see irrelevant matter, the marker will as well. Check that your references are accurate, and then print out your work. Check all the pages. Are they in the right order? Has the printer worked on every page? Now place them in your folder and submit.

6.7 Reading logs

The example in the box was submitted as part of a portfolio of practice evidence from a first-year module. The student has shown what the article was trying to convey, and how it relates to her practice. You may be given such headings. If not, it is important to develop your own, to give your work structure.

Reading log

Full details of publications for referencing purposes:

Kisiel M and Perkins C (2006) Nursing observations: knowledge to help prevent critical illness *British Journal of Nursing* **15** (19): 1052–1056.

What was the article trying to convey?

The article highlights the importance of taking correct observations, particularly in understanding the significance of any changes, and comprehending physiological processes that change the vital signs. To enable nurses to lead with a problem-solving approach and then be able to communicate effectively to other professionals. It goes on to explain the early warning signs of a potentially life-threatening episode, which include changes in pulse, blood pressure, respiratory rate, urine output, temperature and oxygen saturation.

The article introduces the use of blood glucose monitoring, as elevated levels may indicate a reaction to stress caused by shock. But interestingly, oxygen saturation levels are not always a sign, as they only indicate the level of oxygen saturation of the haemoglobin and not how well tissues are being perfused.

By using a case scenario it demonstrates effectively how the body uses compensatory mechanisms to maintain homeostasis, and the signs to look for, both individually but perhaps more particularly as a whole.

How does this relate to your experience/practice?

This article has helped reiterate the importance of taking a patient's observations accurately and consistently, particularly post-operatively. Personally it highlights the need of greater understanding of all the physiological processes and how they work together and compensate for each other.

I also am beginning to appreciate that I will need to develop a problem-solving approach to clinical practice, rather than just data collection, and that I would then be better equipped to communicate information to other professionals more efficiently. I have learnt to communicate with the patient if changes occur to gain additional information, i.e. are they anxious, in pain or have become confused or agitated?

6.8 **Literature review**

You may be asked to select a topic or be given one. You must then search the databases to establish what is already known about the topic. The student below chose to investigate 'Challenging Behaviour associated with Dementia'.

She explains how she did this: 'I searched four nursing-related databases; CINAHL, BNI, MEDLINE, PsychINFO. Table 6.1 shows some of my results. There were lots more'.
Here is a snippet of some of her findings:

Allen and Burns (1995) revealed that at some point 90% of older people with dementia will develop significant behavioural problems, and these manifestations have been found to impact heavily on caregivers (Cohen et al. 1997; Duffy 2003; Robinson et al. 2001).

Name of catalogue, database, subject gateway, or search engine	Key word searches conducted	Results of search (e.g. books and articles located)	Date of search	Limits
CINAHL, BNI, MEDLINE	'Dementia' and 'Older Adults' and 'Challenging Behaviour'	3	16/11/09	(2004–09) Peer-reviewed. linked full text.

Table 6.1 Some results of a nursing database search.

6.9 **Examinations**

Examination conditions in a university are followed strictly. This means no communication of any sort between the candidates, who will be sitting some distance apart. There will be at least two invigilators to ensure that cheating does not occur.

Examinations must demonstrate your knowledge of the subjects, the underpinning theory behind them and their application to practice. How you approach these depends on what is going to be asked of you.

In a 'seen' or 'open-book' examination, you will have time to prepare beforehand. Follow the guidelines you are given. Work out the time you will have to answer the questions. If you are allowed to take books into the exam, only take those you know will help and to which you can quickly refer to what you need to know.

With multiple-choice questions (MCQs), your task is to select the one correct answer from the number of answers offered (see the online resource for more examples of how to approach these).

6.10 **Learning from your marker's feedback**

Once you have received your mark and been successful there is an understandable tendency to want to put the work behind you and focus on the next task. This is a mistake that many students make. You can learn a great deal from reading the marker's comments, both on your script (if your university permits markers to write on it) and on the feedback sheet. Note where it says you have done well; also where you have made errors. Try to build on the areas of success in your next assignment and concentrate on eliminating any errors. Marking feedback in the first year is often quite detailed, correcting errors and putting students on the 'right track' to success. Use this to help you succeed and eliminate errors.

You have not been successful—what now?

Obviously you are going to be disappointed and also possibly cross with yourself. Alternatively, you may feel like blaming the marker or anyone but yourself. These are not unusual reactions. However, indulging in them for too long is unhelpful. You must focus on what you have to do to retrieve this situation as quickly as possible. What happens next depends on two things:

* Whether the failed assignment was your first attempt, second attempt (often known as a retrieval) or a third attempt.
* The rules governing such matters at your university.

First attempt at an assignment: referral (failure)

It would be unusual not to get an automatic second attempt. It is essential that you find out the date that you must submit the second attempt. Do not expect to receive a letter or for anyone to come to you with this information.

The next task is to re-read your original work as soon as you get it back, noting the areas where you have gone wrong. If you have only failed by a few percentage points, it may just be a matter of correcting the areas identified and resubmitting. If you have failed by a larger margin, the task will be greater. The worst-case scenario is that you will have to do a complete re-write of your work. Sometimes lecturers run second-attempt tutorial groups or a 1:1 tutorial. Find what help is available to you and use it. Also use the comments made on the feedback sheet.

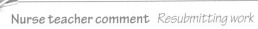

Nurse teacher comment   *Resubmitting work*

66 Make sure you correctly resubmit your work. For instance, check whether you must submit just the new work or also include your first attempt. Do not forget to put on a new top sheet indicating that this is a retrieval submission. Do not miss the final date for submission or you will lose this important second-attempt opportunity. 99

Second-attempt: referral (failure)

You may be given a third attempt, but there is no guarantee. Find out as soon as you can what the position is for you. Do not make any assumptions about your situation from what happens to other students in the same predicament at this time. It may be that your university permits each student one third attempt in each year. If you have not needed a third attempt before, you may get it this time. Others may have used this facility earlier. If you are eligible for a third attempt, you may be told by letter. If you can have a third attempt, you must seek advice and guidance. Note that at some universities you may have to pay to repeat the module and the assessment.

Third attempt: (failure)

Usually a failed third attempt means you being asked to leave the programme. Assessments exist to provide a benchmark of competence. If you have tried three times and failed you must ask yourself if you have the ability to succeed however determined you may be. You may not be able to manage the academic work, but be good practically.

There may well be a role for you should you wish to remain in healthcare. Seek advice from your personal tutor.

Appealing against programme termination

If you feel there are circumstances that have adversely affected your ability to succeed, or you feel you may have grounds for believing you have been treated unfairly, then you need to find out how to appeal. Seek advice from the NUS at your uni. Appeals are not necessarily successful. If reinstated you would almost certainly have to re-join a later cohort.

Summary

This chapter has given you the information and advice you need to be successful in the theory part of the programme. As well as advising you in your study skills, it has highlighted that success is most likely if you submit a good first attempt of your assignment on time. Many of the skills you have read about will be valuable when you go into practice (reading, note-taking, writing, etc.) From now build on these skills and the knowledge you have; take this information with you as you move on to the next chapter, which has been written to smooth your path into clinical practice.

■ Top tips

- Read about essay writing, numeracy, examination tips, etc. before you tackle any of these for real. There is lot of good advice to put you on the right tracks.
- Follow your university guidelines for submissions meticulously.
- Focus your energy where you can get the best marks (see the grading criteria).
- Submission dates and times are rigid—1 second late is too late!
- Submit your work well before the due date time every time.
- Practice helps with your writing and numbers.
- Develop good reading and studying habits.

■ Online resource centre

So you've read about study skills, now you can develop real practical skills! The online resources for this chapter at **www.oxfordtextbooks.co.uk/orc/hart/** include (and will direct you to) lots of advice on study skills and academic work, including guidance, technical help and exercises, all of which will help you to develop the study skills you need for success. You may find it helpful to read these straightaway.

■ References

Barrett D, Wilson B and Woollands A (2009) *Care planning for nurses.* Pearson Education, London.

Buzan T (1993) *The mind map book.* London, BBC.

Giminez J (2007) *Writing for nursing and midwifery students.* Palgrave, Basingstoke.

■ Further reading

Shihab P (2009) *Numeracy in nursing and healthcare; calculations and practice.* Pearson Education, Harlow, Essex.

■ Answers

Answers to numeracy self–assessment

1. 128
2. 4417
3. 14
4. 4
5. 2.7
6. 2.3g
7. 0.3 l. You must always compare like with like, so to covert litres into millilitres you need to multiply by 1000: 0.3 x 1000 = 300. 300 ml is more than 40ml.
8. 70. Add all the ages together = 280, then divide by the number of patients, 4.

Answers to practice based drug calculations

1. Answer = 2

   First of all you need to convert grams to milligrams. There are 1000 milligrams in a gram, therefore the patient needs 2 x 500-mg tablets to equal 1000 mg.

2. Answer = 2.5 ml

   Divide 125 mg by what we want, which is 62.5 mg.

   This = 0.5.

   Then multiply 0.5 by 5.

   Answer = 2.5.

3. Answer = 7.5 ml

   We need 300 mg. If there are 200 mg in 5 ml, there must be 100 mg in 2.5 ml.

   To get 300 mg, multiple 2.5 ml by 3 = 7.5 ml.

4. Answer = 2

   We know this one is easy; the important thing here is to be sure you understand the working out.

Student nurse placements: the big picture

Sue Hart

The aims of this chapter are:

➤ To introduce healthcare, social care and non-statutory health and social care provision

➤ To explain how these sectors work together to support patients and clients

➤ To show how these can be the venues for first-year student nurse clinical placements

The NMC require first-year students to spend about half their time learning in clinical practice settings. You may anticipate that all your placements will be in an NHS hospital setting, after all you are studying to be a nurse and that is where nurses normally work, isn't it? In fact many nurses now work in community settings, residential services, hospices, GP practices or 'walk-in' clinics. Furthermore, a lot of nurses no longer work in the NHS but for a variety of other organizations.

This chapter will explain the variety of contexts in which your practice will take place. Also, it demonstrates through scenarios, how health and social care work together to improve the well-being of patients and clients. We have placed more information about services in Wales, Scotland and Northern Ireland at the online resource.

Important note

This chapter cannot explain *exactly* where you will go for your placements and the precise experiences you will have. This will vary according to your university and the local services available to provide the experiences you need to have.

Student comment

❝I was placed in a home run by a charitable foundation, for 5 adults who had learning disabilities. Although I didn't know it at the time I learnt an awful lot from this placement. I had to learn to how to talk to the clients, all of whom had their own communication styles. The placement definitely was an eye opener to me and looking back was probably one of the best ones I have had in my time as a student.❞

❝ A resident I met in a privately run nursing home was admitted to hospital, and it turned out she was on the medical ward that I was due to go to for my next placement. She was still there when I started on the ward. It was nice to be able to look after her in the home and then in the hospital setting. I was able to take part in the team meetings and I could comment on how she seemed to be recovering, as I had known her before. ❞

! Fact box

Statutory services, such as the NHS and Local Authorities, are mainly funded through taxation (e.g. national insurance, council tax) and are often referred to as 'public sector' services. *Statutory* means 'enacted by statute', i.e. by law, and therefore there is a *legal obligation* to provide the services.

7.1 The National Health Service in the United Kingdom

The NHS employs many people in hundreds of different roles and work areas. In England it employs more than 1.3 million people, in Scotland 158,000, in Wales 71,000 and in

! Fact box

In 2008 the NHS, on average, dealt with approximately one million patients every 36 hours. That is equivalent to 463 people a minute or almost 8 a second (see **www.nhs.uk/aboutnhs**).

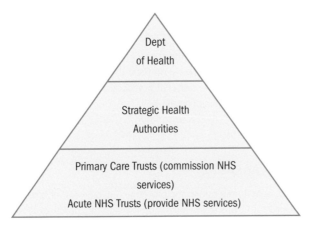

Figure 7.1 Basic structure of the NHS

Northern Ireland 67,000. Almost 50% of NHS employees are clinically qualified; the largest group of these being nurses (approximately 400,000). Additionally, there are in the region of 90,000 hospital doctors, 35,000 general practitioners (GPs) and 16,000 ambulance staff. It is a very complex organization and very expensive—the budget for 2007/2008 exceeded £90 billion (**www.nhs.uk/aboutnhs**).

How is the National Health Service organized?

Figure 7.1 shows the current *basic structure* of the NHS. Since devolution, the NHS in England, Wales, Northern Ireland and Scotland have been managed separately. However, they are still regarded as being part of one unified system. There are some differences across the services in the four countries, but these are outweighed by the similarities.

At the apex of the triangle you can see the Department of Health (DH). The department funds and directs the work of the NHS. The Department of Health website (**www.doh.gov.uk**) is an excellent resource for finding out about NHS policy, and guidelines for practice.

There are ten Strategic Health Authorities (SHAs) in England: North East, North West, Yorkshire and the Humber, East Midlands, East of England, West Midlands, London, South East Coast, South Central and South West. These are responsible for managing the local NHS and communicating with NHS organizations and the DH.

Primary Care Trusts receive about 80% of the NHS budget. They ensure there are sufficient health services in their area to provide for the needs of the local community. They purchase general practitioner (GP) services, dentistry, pharmacy, physiotherapy, podiatry, walk-in centres, etc., as well as commissioning the acute health services with their local NHS Trusts.

+··

Exercise 7.1

If you do not already know it, find out the name of the PCT in the area where you will be doing your placements. Visit their website and see the sorts of services they purchase on behalf of the local community. How many GP practices are there in your area? Is NHS dentistry available? Are there any special hospitals?

···

> ! **Fact box**
>
> Primary Care Trusts once had a role in the provision (i.e. delivery) of direct patient or client services. They are currently moving to just a commissioning/purchasing role.

Acute NHS Trusts services may be provided in local general hospitals, outpatient departments, hospital or community-based clinics or in the homes of patients and clients.

At the time of writing in England there are 12 *NHS Ambulance Trusts* and, with their counterparts the Scottish, Welsh and Northern Ireland ambulance services, provide emergency access to healthcare. The NHS must also ensure that patients who have mobility problems, or who are old or infirm, can get to hospital for non-emergency appointments.

Mental Health Trusts provide health and social care services for people with mental health problems. If someone is depressed (e.g. after a bereavement) they may seek help from their GP. If they do not improve after initial treatment they may be referred to a psychiatrist.

Special Health Authorities provide a specialist health service to the whole country (e.g. England) and not just to a local community, e.g. Blood Service (see **www.nationalblood.co.uk**).

Special Hospitals provide expert treatment that can be accessed by patients from all parts of the country, e.g. the National Spinal Injuries Centre (NSIC) (see **www.spinal.org.uk**) at Stoke Mandeville Hospital in Buckinghamshire.

NHS Foundation Trusts have been in existence since April 2004. One attraction is the enhanced financial and operational freedom that comes with its Foundation status.

How do patients and clients access the NHS?

Figure 7.2 shows the different levels of NHS provision available for patients and clients. Be careful not to confuse Primary Care with Primary Care Trusts.

Primary Care is the first point of contact with the NHS for most patients and has its main focus on health, as opposed to illness. General practitioner (GP) services are based in primary care. Most non-emergency referrals (also known as *planned admissions*) to secondary care are made by the patient's GP.

Secondary Care refers to the services provided by the NHS acute trusts outlined above. Anyone on a waiting list for surgery will go to hospital as a planned admission.

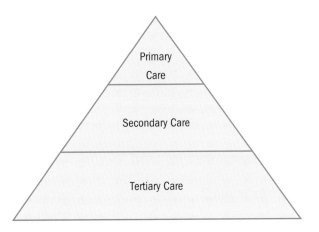

Figure 7.2 Levels of NHS provision available for patients and clients

Tertiary Care refers to the highly specialized care provided by special hospitals (such as the NSIC referred to above). Patients access tertiary care from secondary care.

An example of a patient's journey in the NHS

When you are in your placement, part of your learning will come from listening to patients' stories, e.g. about their ill health and admission. Was their admission planned or an emergency? Is this their first episode of depression?

The following gives you an example of a patient journey through each level of the NHS, and how they get the care they need.

✚

Nursing practice example 1

Elaine is a 28-year-old teacher. Her job is stressful and she often rushes lunch. Yesterday she noticed blood in her stools. As her brother has had colon cancer, Elaine is aware that this symptom can be serious. She is also aware that there could be other causes for it. After two weeks the situation persists and she goes to her GP. Doctor Kagee refers Elaine to her local hospital for a colonoscopy. This reveals a number of pre-cancerous polyps, which are removed. There are also a number of growths that could be seen but were difficult to remove. Mr Logan, the Consultant, refers Elaine to St. Mark's in Harrow, the national centre for bowel cancer. Elaine has two further colonoscopies at St Mark's. The treatment successfully removes all sign of the growths.

Primary care: GP

Secondary care: Acute NHS Trust

Tertiary/specialist care: St. Mark's Hospital Harrow (**www.stmarksfoundation.org**).

Nursing practice example 2

Mavis, aged 78, needs a hip replacement. Her GP referred her to the hospital when she complained of pain, reduced mobility and difficulty sleeping due to discomfort. As it was a non-urgent case, Mavis attended the outpatient clinic. On the same day she had an X-ray. It was decided to perform the hip-replacement surgery as soon as possible. A bed was booked and Mavis received a letter at home advising her of the admission date.

Primary care: GP

Secondary care: Admission to orthopaedic ward, Acute NHS Trust

Nursing practice example 3

Harry has been depressed since the death of his wife a year ago. He has stopped self-caring to the point of neglect and has started drinking a bottle of vodka a day. Harry has agreed to let a community psychiatric nurse, Sally, visit him at home. Sally is shocked at Harry's self-neglect. Her concerns increase when Harry says that the tinned food in his store cupboard has been poisoned and that if he eats it, he fears he will die. He says he would rather end it all, than let *them* kill him. Sally makes an emergency referral to a psychiatrist.

Primary care: GP

Secondary care: NHS Mental Health Trust

7.2 Social care provision

Although you are studying to be a nurse, you need to understand about social care provision because:

- many patients and clients receive services from both the health and social care sectors, so you need to understand how the system works;

- many NHS Trusts deliver health *and* social care services—some employ nurses as well as social carers (e.g. case managers);

- it is *possible* that during your time as a student nurse you will be sent to at least one placement in the social care sector.

Background

The statutory provision of social care is primarily the responsibility of the local authority (local council) area in which the person lives. A goal of social care is to enable people to live as independently as possible in their own homes, or alternatively to live well in a residential service or other supported environment. It is often the most vulnerable people in society who require social care support, e.g. older people, or those who have been in hospital, those with a physical, sensory or learning disability, or a chronic physical or mental health problem (for more see **www.dh.gov.uk/en/SocialCare/Aboutthedirectorate/Howsocialcareisdelivered/index.htm**).

Examples of why social care support may be needed

Social carers perform a variety of tasks to meet the individual's needs. This could range from making food and hot drinks, to cleaning, shopping and assisting the person to get washed and dressed. They help in situations as follows:

- Where someone is unable to carry out essential self-care or domestic routines, e.g. preparing drinks.
- If abuse has been reported or there are concerns that it may occur.
- If a person has multiple and chronic health problems.
- If someone is homeless or likely to be made homeless.
- Where carers are no longer able to cope.
- If the care network is at risk of collapse or no longer being well supported by others.

Exercise 7.2

If you do not already know it, find out the name of the Local Authority in the area where you will be doing your placements. Visit their website. What social care services do they offer for children and their families, disabled people and the homeless?

How do patients and clients access social care?

This will depend on individual circumstances. Let's go back to Mavis (above). The hip-replacement surgery was successful and she began mobilizing (i.e. walking again slowly) within a couple of days. She was keen to get home, although the nurses caring for her were not sure that this was wise. They felt Mavis needed to be seen at home regularly for the first week, to be certain she was safe.

A multi-disciplinary discharge planning meeting was held where Mavis' circumstances were discussed with her. It was agreed that she could go home soon and that social care support workers would visit every day for the first week and then twice a week after that, to help Mavis in the bath.

• • • A word about Care packages

The various elements of care needed to support a person are known collectively as the *care package*. When future care needs will be funded by a PCT (e.g. a place in a registered care home), a continuing care nurse assessor will see the patient. The assessor will consider the care package being proposed, to ensure it is value for money and the best option for the person. If a patient is self-funded, this assessment will not be necessary.

> **! Fact box** Safeguarding adults and children
>
> NHS Trust and Local Authorities have 'safeguarding teams' who have a special remit to prevent the abuse of vulnerable people, and intervene where abuse has occurred. Abuse comes in many forms: discriminatory, financial, neglect, physical, psychological, verbal.

Other routes into social care support could be any of the following:

- The police may involve social care services if they were asked to see an older person in an A&E department with unexplained bruising on their body.
- A family member may contact social care services directly to request home care support for an elderly person.
- A person who lives alone who has developed multiple sclerosis and is now a wheelchair user. She has an adapted car and can work but needs help to wash and dress in the morning.

Those applying to receive social care will have a needs assessment done by the local authority. The law allows local authorities to decide what to charge for social care services, as long as it is not more than the services cost to provide.

Exercise 7.3

Find out about your local safeguarding teams. Look at the NHS Trust and Local Authority websites. See the DH website for the 'No secrets' guidance (2000) and read 'Every child matters' (2003) (**www.everychildmatters.gov.uk/publications**). Raise your awareness that abuse happens; know about safeguarding.

Exercise 7.4

Why might Harry (above) need social care services for some time after his discharge from hospital? Can you think if Elaine would need such services?

7.3 Voluntary sector health and social care provision (3rd sector)

As well as the two *statutory* sectors (health and social care) described above, there are numerous organizations that play an important role in health and social care but which are *not* funded directly out of taxation and National Insurance. There is no statutory duty to provide these services and citizens have no statutory right to receive them.

These are usually funded by a mixture of donations, subscriptions, legacies and a variety of other fund-raising activities. Some have paid employees, others unpaid volunteers, many have a mixture of both.

The activities of voluntary organizations are summarized below, with many being involved in one or more of the following:

- Influencing policy.
- Supporting services.
- Campaigning.
- Raising awareness.
- Promoting service standards.

Some voluntary sector services have worked in health and social care for a long time. For example, Mencap for people with learning disabilities; Age Concern for older people; Mind, for those with mental health needs. Child Line offers advice to children and young people who are worried.

Earlier you will have read that PCTs commission services on behalf of the local population. It is often from the voluntary sector that such services are bought. An example could be a housing association working alongside a Mental Health NHS Trust to provide homes for people with long-term mental ill health needs.

7.4 **Private or independent sector services**

Student comment

66 I had a privately owned nursing home placement first. It was good for me because I had not worked as a **healthcare assistant**, so felt a bit daunted about going to a hospital ward. I had a chance to learn and become comfortable with personal care and manual handling. I now really value doing this on the wards because I have seen it is a way to become close to patients and build trusting relationships. 99

Some health and social care provision is provided by private firms, such as independently owned registered residential care homes or nursing homes for older people. Some of these operate on a 'not-for-profit' basis, meaning that any money made over and above that needed to pay the staff and deliver the service is put back into the firm. Others are for profit, delivering services as a business to make money.

+ ··

Exercise 7.5

What are some of the non-statutory services or private services working in your area? Find what services exist for older people, people with learning disability or physical disability, or those with a mental health need. Are there any specialist children's services?

··

7.5 **How do patients and clients access non-statutory services?**

Again, this will depend on individual circumstances. If they wish to receive them, patients, clients and their families must pay for a non-statutory service. For example:

- An older person may prefer to pay to live in a private nursing home.

- A person who is anxious may pay privately for a counsellor to help them.

+ ··

Nursing practice example 4

Mavis and Harry both received social care services for some time after they were discharged from hospital. Harry had a social care support worker calling in every day for the first 2 weeks after he was home to ensure that he was self-caring. Sometimes the support worker accompanied Harry to the local shop to buy food.

   Can you now think of any non-statutory health and social care services that Mavis or Harry may benefit from?

   Mavis decided to pay for herself to have a weekly visit to an acupuncturist, as she believes this may speed up her recovery.

   Harry realizes that his alcohol consumption was becoming a problem. He finds out about 'Alcoholics Anonymous' (AA) and is going to his first meeting next week.

··

7.6 **The 'mixed economy of care'**

When health and social care is on the one hand provided by the state, but also on the other provided by charities, private firms and voluntary sector organizations, it can get very complicated; this phrase (DH 1989) seeks to capture that complexity. When you unpick it you can see that it says that there are various (mixed) funding streams (economy) and services that are available to ensure that patients and clients get the help and support (care) they need.

> ! **Fact box** Commissioning services
>
> When the public sector buys services from the private sector, this is known as *commissioning* or *purchasing* services. For example, most cleaning services in acute hospital settings are delivered by privately managed and run companies.

> · · · **A word about** Community
>
> You will hear the term community care, but what does it mean? Community is used in many contexts, e.g:
>
> - local community (can mean all the people who live in area);
> - community or cottage hospital (small local hospital with no A&E department);
> - local community (can mean the actual place e.g. university community);
> - gay community; shared interest;
> - collective community of car owners; common ownership;
> - community 'at large', i.e. the general public;
> - community enterprise (e.g. shared working on a project);
> - faith communities (Buddhist, Roman Catholic, Jewish, i.e. linked by religious belief);
> - minority ethnic community (linked by ethnic background).
>
> In relation to health and social care, the term community care is so broad that it now basically means care that does not take place in an acute or special hospital trust.

Ideally you now have a basic knowledge of health and social care provision. This is necessary if you are to understand how your first year placements are organized. The rest of this chapter will consider these issues.

7.7 How first-year student nurse clinical placements are organized

You will now have a basic understanding of where patients and clients get the care and treatment they need. They get a lot of this from the NHS but also from the other areas outlined. For this reason many non-NHS institutions such as special schools, social services departments and charities e. g. Mencap are used as placements for student nurses. As the student comments have shown, these can be very rich and valuable learning experiences.

Student comment

❝ The non-NHS placement I had in the CFP was a privately owned residential home for people with neuro-type probs, but consisted of a large group of people with Huntington's Disease (HD). The manager was extremely knowledgeable about the condition and was passionate about giving the best possible care and quality of life to the clients. All the HD patients were part of a study and attended regular appointments at UCL (University College London) and sometimes I was able to accompany them for this. I was also lucky enough to attend a lecture and a tour of the Royal Hospital for Neuro Disabilities as part of HD awareness week. I felt privileged to be a part of this and it also provided me with an interesting insight into a disease that I knew nothing about before the placement, but was to prove invaluable in the next placement, as I met a lady with HD who had been placed in a dementia unit. I felt that my knowledge of her illness exceeded that of the staff that had not cared for anyone with HD. ❞

Education audit

For a placement area to be considered a suitable learning environment it must have gone through an education audit. This is an NMC requirement and applies to all settings outside, as well as within, the NHS. It confirms:

- The learning experiences and quality of support available for students.
- The standard practice in the placement (is it evidence-based and up-to-date?).
- The facilities available conducive to learning?
- The necessary support to the placement and mentor (e.g. through the liaison tutor role).

Nurse teacher comment

❝ From time to time I have had students in X or Y placements say 'there is nothing to learn here'. Of course they do not realize that the link tutor has done an education audit and confirmed what learning can occur there. I explain to the student that, of course there are learning opportunities; it is just *whether they can see them* . . . . I see it as part of my role to help a student to make this connection. ❞

Summary

This chapter has helped you to understand the sorts of placements you can expect to have in the first year, by walking you through some of the services available to patient and clients. Although most placements occur in NHS settings, it is important to value the opportunities that may come your way to experience an independent or social care environment. It is less likely that you will have such experiences later in the programme, so make the most of them now.

■ Top tips

- Value your learning opportunities outside NHS placements.
- You do not just learn on a *ward in your uniform.*
- You do not have to be busy and rushing around to be learning.
- Find out what others do, nurses do not work in isolation.
- Find out as much as you can about the services available in your area.
- Understanding how the health, social care and other sectors work will assist your future practice and reference to this in your assignments would suggest you have a more fully rounded understanding of the caring professions.
- Never see a patient or client as a set of *conditions* or an *illness*. They are unique individuals with various needs; that is why the range of services above exist.

■ Online resource centre

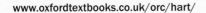 Health and social care is organized in different ways throughout the UK and directions to key websites are provided online for readers in Scotland, Northern Ireland and Wales. Charity websites including 'Mencap', 'Mind', and 'Age Concern' are a great place to get more information on how you can improve the well-being of patients and clients. For weblinks to these charities, and more information on social care, go online to: **www.oxfordtextbooks.co.uk/orc/hart/**

■ References

Department of Health (1989) *Caring for people: community care in the next decade and beyond.* HMSO, London.

■ Further reading

Adams R (2007) *Foundations of health and social care.* Palgrave Macmillan, Basingstoke Hampshire.

■ Websites

About NHS Choices: **http://www.nhs.uk/aboutNHSChoices/Pages/AboutNHSChoices.aspx**

Department of Health: **http://www.dh.gov.uk/en/index.htm**

The National Blood Service for England and North Wales: **http://www.blood.co.uk/**

The Royal Marsden NHS Foundation Trust: **http://www.royalmarsden.nhs.uk/rmh**

Royal Hospital for Neuro-disability: **http://www.rhn.org.uk/**

Department of Health, Social Services and Public Safety, Northern Ireland: **http://www.dhsspsni. gov.uk/**

Department of Health information about how social care is delivered: **http://www.dh.gov.uk/en/ SocialCare/Aboutthedirectorate/Howsocialcareisdelivered/index.htm**

Preparing you for clinical practice

Debbie Roberts

The aims of this chapter are:

➤ To introduce how placements are organized and how to find out what you need to know

➤ To introduce some of the ways you will be prepared to go into your first placements

➤ To suggest what you can do to make your journey into practice a smooth one

This chapter will help to build your confidence by outlining the variety of ways nurse teachers prepare students before they first go into practice. It would be unusual not to have a first-year clinical placement experience in your own future field of practice and often in the other fields as well. However, you need to accept that this broad experience may not always be possible. For example, it is highly unlikely, wherever you are studying, that every student will experience a child or paediatric ward, due to the limited availability of such placements. Also, placements in learning disabilities services are not always available.

8.1 Placements: the basics you will be told

First-year student nurse clinical placements are normally allocated for students by placement officers employed specifically for this role. It is these support staff who make all the arrangements, in collaboration with the nurse teachers and colleagues in the placements.

You will be told as far in advance as possible where you will be going and how to find out the information you need. It may be posted on a notice board or student website (or both). You need to know from the university:

- The dates of the placement.
- The address and telephone number of where you are going.
- Whether it is an adult, child, learning disability or mental health experience.
- The name of your mentor or the person to contact if this is different.
- The telephone number/email for your mentor.

It helps to remember, that the placement office staff deal with hundreds of different placement areas. They will ensure you have the basic information in the bullet points above, but it has to be *your* responsibility to make contact and find out the finer details about your placement. You can do this by telephoning or by arranging to call in, at a time suitable for the placement. You are encouraged to make contact with the placement in good time before you start as this enables you:

- To find out the best way to get there.
- If you are going to drive, to find out where to park. Will you need to pay?
- To find out what time to arrive on the first day.
- To know what to take with you.
- To know what to wear.

(See Chapter 10 for more information about your first steps into practice.)

Nurse teacher comment *Getting to your future placement*

"Placements officers know where you live and if you have your own transport, and take this into account when allocating placements. However, if you foresee significant problems getting to the placement you have been allocated, then make your concern known to the placement officer or your personal tutor, in plenty of time before you are due to start. But, before you do this, see **www.transportdirect.co.uk** to find public transport options. Directions to drive are available from the Automobile Association (AA) website **www.theaa.com/route-planner**. All you need is the postcode of your starting point and your destination."

8.2 **Changing placements**

Some universities will not allow you to change your placements because of the potential problems of twenty students all wanting to attend one particular placement at the same time. Others are more flexible and may allow you an element of choice. Some might even expect you to negotiate your own placements from a list. Basically, the particular process of allocating students to placements varies a little from university to university. If you do wish to change, you need to find out how to do this. It sometimes can help your request to change if there is a student who would agree to a direct swap with you (e.g. adult placement for adult placement for the same number of weeks). If you ask to swap, you must provide good reasons and be prepared to be disappointed most of the time.

8.3 **How nurse teachers prepare students for clinical practice**

Rest assured that long before you first go into any placements as a first-year student your nurse teachers will have started preparing you for that experience. They need to be satisfied that, before you meet any member of the public, you are equipped with the essential knowledge, skills and (hopefully) confidence to enter safely into practice, under the supervision of your mentor. All universities are different but the following outlines some of the ways we know that this pre-placement preparation occurs.

Preparing you for clinical practice 1: skills laboratories and simulated settings

Before going out into clinical practice you will be taught some of the essential skills in the safe and non-threatening setting of a skills laboratory or skills room. These are rooms that are usually set up like a ward or clinical area but without real patients. Here you will be taught a variety of skills, some (not all!) of which you will practice on your fellow students. These sessions are sometimes taught by nurse lecturers, or by nurses who will come into the university from practice.

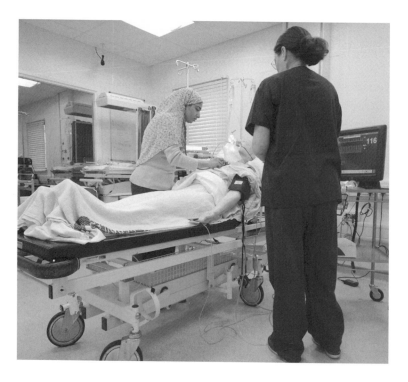

Figure 8.1 Students in a skills laboratory with permission of Alex Rawlings, OxSim Centre

Uniform

To give an authentic feel to practice, and to help adult and child nurses get used to being in uniform, many universities ask for full and correct uniform to be worn in the skills lab. If so, read your university guidelines for exactly what they want. It is likely to include the following basics:

- nail polish is removed;
- rings other than a wedding band are removed;
- certain piercings may need to be removed (discuss with your personal tutor);
- long hair is tied back;
- wrist watches are removed;
- regulation shoes are worn;
- certain tattoos, which are visible below the elbow, may need to be covered (if relevant it is a good idea to discuss this with your personal tutor *before* you go into practice).

If mufti (non-uniform) is permitted in the skills lab you may be directed to wear loose, comfortable clothing, especially if doing manual handling. (See more about appearance in Chapter 14.)

> ! **Fact box** Uniform
>
> You will have been advised about obtaining your uniform long before you go into practice for the first time. If you have not yet done so, you may be expected to purchase your own uniform from a specific shop. In some cases the cost of this is reimbursed to you on the production of a receipt, up to an agreed maximum sum (e.g. up to £70 value of uniform). In such cases, if you want more than two tunics, you might have to buy them yourself. Other universities contract with a supplier who will come and measure you and then later deliver your uniforms. Universities tend only to provide uniforms at the start of the programme, so if you gain or lose weight (unexpectedly or otherwise), you might have to buy your own better fitting uniforms further on in the programme.

Skills lab sessions

These will usually involve:

- An explanation of the underpinning theory. This means an explanation is given about when and why the skill would be needed. It will probably also include links back to a lecture you have had on the topic.
- A demonstration by the teacher of the skill to be learned.
- You being given the opportunity under supervision to practice the skill.

> ! **Fact box** How you would learn hand washing in a skills lab
>
> First the teacher may stress the many reasons why it is so important that nurses wash their hands frequently, e.g before and after giving nursing care to *every* patient. To aid your understanding of the theory/practice links, they may refer back to lectures you have had on microbiology and infection control. They will then demonstrate the correct method of hand-washing. Later you will be given the opportunity to practice this skill under supervision, with the teacher correcting any errors you make until you are confident. (See Chapter 5 for a reminder of theory/practice links, if you are still unsure of this term.)

Activities you might cover in the skills labs in your first year

- Hand-washing (one of the most important clinical skills you will learn), as well as infection control and the principles of asepsis (i.e. the absence of harmful bacteria).
- Moving and handling means how to move patients and equipment safely. You would not be permitted or be safe to go into practice without having learnt this essential skill beforehand.
- Handling wheelchairs.
- Cardio-pulmonary resuscitation, also known as basic life support, is provided when someone stops breathing or their heart stops beating unexpectedly.
- Communication and interpersonal skills. This sounds straightforward, but like any other skill it requires practice. Good communication skills are the cornerstone of nursing.

- Bed-bathing, washing and helping someone to wash and skin care.

- Oral hygiene, to clean teeth and mouth using toothbrush and paste or other methods.

- Positioning for comfort and pressure sore prevention.

- Helping someone to eat and drink at a table, when they are bed-bound or have sensory or physical disabilities.

- Helping someone with elimination needs. This means helping a patient to use a lavatory or provide them with a bedpan, commode chair or bottle. It can also involve caring for patients with indwelling urinary catheters and the giving of suppositories and enemas. (Don't worry, you will not have to practice giving these to each other!)

- Injection techniques—subcutaneous and intramuscular.

- Taking and recording vital signs and other measurements: blood pressure, pulse, respiration, temperature, fluid balance.

- Bed-making and adjusting, both with patient and empty.

The clinical skills labs are an ideal place to rehearse and practise your skills in a safe and non-threatening environment. Nursing is a practical discipline and you will need to learn a whole range of psychomotor skills—these are movements performed, as a result of conscious mental activity, most often with the hands, e.g. giving an injection.

Learning these skills takes time, and as a learner you are at first allowed to make mistakes; to do so is understandable. Learning in the skills lab means that you can make mistakes and learn from them, *before* you practice on *real* patients. The skills lab is a really useful place to learn, particularly at the beginning of your course, and it will help you integrate classroom theory and clinical practice.

Preparing you for clinical practice 2: simulated learning

This refers to the *type of learning* that takes place in the skills laboratory. In other words that simulated learning in a skills lab *imitates* practice. The skills are practised on fellow students or mannequins (not patients) in skills labs (not wards or units). The NMC (2007) allow 'up to a maximum of 300 hours to be used to provide clinical training within a simulated practice learning environment in support of providing direct care in the practice setting'. Ideally many of these hours will be used before you go into practice for the first time.

Some universities may choose to use other methods of teaching you some of these essential nursing skills and make use of virtual learning environments and computer software to help you to learn. These will also take you through a *clinical encounter* (i.e. nurse giving footcare to a patient with diabetes) in a step-by-step fashion, providing you with demonstrations and asking you questions to ensure that you have understood and learned from the experience. You may also come across special mannequins (dummies) that can be programmed to produce a range of realistic symptoms, including vomiting, bleeding and respiratory problems.

Preparing you for clinical practice 3: observed structured clinical examination (OSCE)

Before going out into clinical practice you may be tested or examined on a range of skills; this examination is known as an 'OSCE'. You will have to perform a skill (such as cardiopulmonary resuscitation) according to a strict protocol; in other words, you will have to do the right things in the right order and demonstrate the correct technique in order to pass the test. OSCE can be used to test a wide range of skills and these can vary according to the university where you study. The advantage of doing the test in a skills lab of course is that you will be using a mannequin rather than real patients, and you can refine your skills until you feel confident and competent. (See the online resource centre for OSCE tips.)

Preparing you for clinical practice 4: NHS Trust introductions

Nurse teacher comment   *Trust allocation*

" Your allocated 'Trust' refers to the main venue where you will be having your placements, and this indicates the general area in which your placements will occur. You may be allocated to an NHS Mental Health Trust for your mental health experience, but also have a placement in a local authority run service in the local town. "

Before starting your placements you may find that the NHS Trust to which you have been allocated will invite you to attend for an induction day, a few days or even a week. Often attendance will be mandatory (i.e. compulsory). Elements covered at Trust induction will vary, but typically you will be given an overview of the Trust, where to find various buildings and departments, information about parking, the uniform guidelines, start and finish times, and the expectations of you as a student. There may be an opportunity for you to meet the managers of directorates or services and the senior nurses who will all explain their role within the organization. In a longer induction you may be introduced to Trust policies and procedures such as infection control, health and safety, manual handling and fire.

Preparing you for clinical practice 5: before your placement starts

As referred to above, before your first day in placement it is considered good professional behaviour (more about this in Chapters 14 and 15) to make a short courtesy visit to the placement in order to introduce yourself to the nurse in charge and your mentor. You must telephone or email beforehand to arrange this, and visit *only when it is convenient* for the staff. Once there, this should only take 5 minutes or so, and can be time well spent. You can find out when to arrive and your 'off-duty' (see below) for the next week. You can ask the nurse in charge to recommend some reading to do beforehand. You might also want to find out how care is organized and whether the placement uses a particular model of nursing.

By visiting you give the impression of being organized, keen and professional. Also, even just being in a placement for a few minutes can help alleviate the 'night before nerves'—often these are about what it will be like. To a degree you can get a 'feel' for an environment in a few minutes. Also, by visiting you give your mentor or the nurse in charge the opportunity to say 'we are looking forward to having you here' and this can make all the difference. If you do not visit before you start, you miss an opportunity for this to happen.

Nurse teacher comment

66 For adult and child nurses especially, note there will be somewhere you can change into your uniform on arrival at your placement. Good to check this out before you go. This university does not permit students to wear their uniform to travel or outside the clinical area. It may be a pain to have to arrive a little earlier to get changed, however when doing my shopping in Sainsbury's at 3.00 p.m. I do not want to see a student in their soiled uniform picking over the apples. Infection control! 99

••• **A word about** 'Off-duty'

In the world of nursing, the term 'off-duty' refers to the rota that shows when you will be on-duty (the days and shift times you will be on the ward or unit) as well as when you will be off-duty (i.e. when your day/days off will be). The 'off-duty' is usually worked out by the nurse in charge. Off-duty might be done in advance for the entire placement, or only a week at a time.

So far, this chapter has talked through some of the *specific sessions* you will have to prepare for, but preparing you for practice will also happen in many others ways. You almost certainly will have a session where a teacher talks through the assessment of practice paperwork. Also you will have had lectures on communication skills, where you will learn about verbal and non-verbal communication, listening, observation and possibly even record-keeping skills. You will have had some introductions to law, ethics and social policy. Care planning will have been covered. You may have had introductory talks about adult, child, learning disability and mental health placements, and what to expect there. Reading Chapter 11 will also add to this.

Remember also that you are intended to take what you have learned so far in formal lectures, in classroom discussions, in conversation with your personal tutor group, and from your own reading, *into the placement with you*. That is the best preparation you can give yourself.

8.4 **Preparing to learn in practice**

Student comment

66 Before you go, if you can, talk to other students who have had a placement there, find out some background about the area and what to expect. Find out what kind of problems and needs the patients on that placement will be experiencing, so you can be prepared, and do some reading up before you start. 99

You must never enter a placement without understanding *why* you are going and *what you need to learn* when there. The next chapter explains how you will learn once you get into practice. Now it is time to prepare the ground for that learning.

Exercise 8.1 Preparing for practice

Promise yourself now that *before you go into practice for the first time* you will read at least Chapters 7, 9, 10 and 11 of this book. Reading Chapter 14 would also be excellent preparation. If you do this, you will understand the context in which you are learning and better understand the field of practice in which you are to gain experience. You will also understand why the NMC require nursing students to have experience in all four fields of practice in the first year.

Also *read all the information you have been given by your nurse teachers* about your forthcoming practice. This information could have come to you from a variety of sources, from several different teachers and support staff, and be in hard copy format or electronic. At this point, if you have followed the filing and sorting tips in Chapter 4, it should all be in one folder for you to read.

Mentor comment

66 Reading through the paperwork is particularly important at the beginning of the course. It takes time to familiarize yourself with the documents and what you need to complete. You need to do this in order that you can be sure you complete all aspects of the assessment correctly. Why put your future assessment of practice success at risk by handing in an incomplete portfolio? 99

66 You may have a mentor who is very experienced and knows the paperwork back to front; it is equally possible that your mentor is new and that you are the first student they are going to have. 99

It is *likely* that the paperwork for your portfolio will consist of the following:

- Professional behaviour sheets.
- Summative (final) assessment of practice.
- Mentor final report on your practice (i.e. to 'sign you off') at the end of the practice.
- Action plan (if required).
- Ongoing record of achievement.
- Observation of your practice record.
- Practice learning outcomes (with space for your mentor and you to make comments and sign).
- Orientation to placement.
- Learning agreements.
- Mentor/co-mentor/associate mentor signature sheets.
- Formative (first) assessment of practice.
- Skills development record.

Record of attendance/time sheet.

- Visits record.
- Short placement record.
- Lists of activities that, as a first-year student nurse, you must not undertake when in practice: the do's and don'ts.
- Paperwork about any additional activities you must perform (such as keeping a reflective journal, submitting reading logs).

It will help you to familiarize yourself with all the paperwork. Chapter 13 will discuss your assessment of practice and what to do with the paperwork.

Mentor comment

66 You may be given all the necessary paperwork for all your first-year practice at one time by your nurse teachers. Alternatively, you may be given it (or have to collect it) for every placement. Make sure you bring everything you have been given on the first day. This way we can check it and, if there is anything missing, you can obtain it in plenty of time before your final assessment. 99

Summary

The above has given you an understanding of how you will be prepared before you start your clinical placements. The next chapter explains some of the ways student nurses can learn in practice.

■ Top tips

- Preparing well for practice will build your confidence.
- Practice wearing your uniform helps you to grow to feel comfortable in it.
- The more you practise essential skills, such as BPs, the more skilled you become.
- Reading the theory behind the nursing skills aids your understanding.
- Keep safe all your records of attendance at the skills lab sessions (for evidence later, if needed).

■ Online resource centre

 You can find tips on how to prepare for clinical practice and succeed in your OSCEs by going online to **www.oxfordtextbooks.co.uk/orc/hart/**

■ References

NMC Circular 36 (2007) *Supporting direct care through simulated practice learning in the pre-registration nursing programme*. NMC, London.

■ Further reading

Barrett D, Wilson B and Woollands A (2009) *Care planning: a guide for nurses*. Pearson Education, Harlow, Essex.

Debnath R (2009) *Professional skills in nursing a guide for the common foundation programme*. Sage, London.

Shihab P (2009) *Numeracy in nursing and healthcare; calculations and practice*. Pearson Education, Harlow, Essex.

Smith J (2005) *The guide to the handling of people* (5th edn). London Backcare in collaboration with the Royal College of Nursing and National Back Exchange.

How you will learn in practice

Debbie Roberts

The aims of this chapter are:

➤ To highlight the many ways student nurses learn in practice

➤ To explore the role of the mentor in practice

➤ To offer guidance about working with your mentor

➤ To help you recognize and maximize learning opportunities

This chapter will explain the ways that student nurses learn in practice and explores the language of learning. It shows that the more you are inquisitive, questioning, interested in and engaged in the activities going on, the more you will learn. When you are *open* to learning, you will see learning opportunities everywhere. As well as from patients and clients, you can learn a lot from senior nurses, doctors, from the ward clerk to the senior consultant, health and social care support workers, home managers, psychologists and physiotherapists. Although it may not be specifically the role of any of these individuals to teach you, simply by observing them and listening you can learn a great deal.

As noted in Chapter 7, in order that your nurse teachers can be confident that you can learn what you need to know (i.e. there are *learning opportunities* available) all placements must have gone through a process known as an education audit. This happens before any students are placed in an area and is an NMC requirement. This chapter starts by illustrating how your learning is supported by your designation, as a student, as '*supernumerary*'.

9.1 What is supernumerary status and why is it important?

Your role as a learner in practice is strengthened by 'supernumerary status'. As a student nurse you do not *go to work* in the way that the professionals and other paid staff do. You go to a placement to 'learn' for a short time and then move to another placement to learn more. In your placement you are of course working as well (e.g. assisting patients, learning nursing procedures, attending case conferences, etc.), but as a student nurse you are there principally to learn *through the work you are doing*.

> ### Mentor comment
>
> ❝ Supernumerary status is *not* a licence simply to observe from the wings, read client notes all day or spend more time on community visits than on the unit. Of course these are important but there must be a balance. Some students I have had came with strange ideas of what they need to do to meet their learning outcomes. How would I explain it? Students learn, under supervision by doing the work assigned to them by their mentor. Sometimes this is hands on; other times by observations and visits, etc. ❞

Supernumerary status means that you are not included in the 'regular' ('established') ward or unit workforce in terms of the hours you will 'work' in practice. Also, you will not be counted as a member of the rostered number of staff on duty and your name will not be on the rota as a member of staff. However, for convenience, and so people know to expect you, your name may be on the rota, that is the staff list. If your name is there it will be *additional* to the regular staff. So, if three registered nurses and five healthcare assistants normally work on the unit, the 'established' staff would be eight. If you are placed there, it should still be eight staff, plus one (you).

Supernumerary status reinforces your role as a learner as opposed to an employee. Prior to the introduction of supernumerary status, student nurses were sometimes used simply to get the work done, often at the expense of their own learning. With supernumerary status, if a member of the team is away then, *as a rule*, a student nurse should not be expected to cover the person's absence. Having said that, if you are in a situation one day where there is a staffing crisis on the ward, it would be considerate of you, under supervision and only working to the level of your own competence, to assist the regular staff to perform the necessary duties. If you are asked routinely to cover for a missing colleague, and this is interfering with your learning, you must draw this to the attention of your mentor or nurse teachers.

> ### Student comment
>
> ❝ I have been used as 'another pair of hands' for a while on my current placement, which has been fine at times, but annoying at others. My way of coping is to arrange as many learning opportunities as possible. So I arranged visits off the ward and if someone came on the ward, like the continuing care nurse, for example, I asked if they could spend some time with me, explaining what they do and why. I also tapped into »

the team's knowledge; one nurse told me she knew all about syringe drivers, so I had some time with her. All the other times I accepted that this was not permanent and that, frustrating as it was to hear my colleagues talking about all the learning opportunities they were getting, while I was on toileting duties, I knew it was only for a short period of time. Soon I would be off to pastures new! **99**

9.2 The language of student nurse learning

As you read through the paperwork you have been given, note some of the terminology that you must now use (e.g. learning agreements). If there is a glossary of terms to help your understanding, *it is a good idea to read this now*. If not, then the following will help. Note that different placements and universities may use other terminology, but many of the terms below are widely used:

- *Goals:* a term used to describe what you want to achieve within a placement.

- *Learning aims:* another way of saying the above.

- *Learning outcomes:* a term used to describe what you will learn throughout the placement. Learning outcomes are defined for you by the practice area and university staff, and the NMC year-one outcomes.

- *Learning need:* is (logically) what you need to learn. These needs may be what the programme dictates (e.g. learning outcomes, as above) or alternatively what you know you need to learn, e.g. your mentor on your last placement voiced some concern about your communication skills and confidence to speak when working with patients. On your *next placement* it would be sensible to identify 'communication skills' and 'confidence-building activities regarding communication' as learning needs in order to focus on this area.

- *Learning experiences:* a term used to describe the total learning that takes place, both formally and informally, within a clinical placement.

- *Learning agreements:* a term used to describe an agreement between you and your mentor, personal teacher or academic link teacher, which specifies the goal to be achieved, a time-frame for the goal to be met; it also details what all parties will be responsible for within the contract (see more in Chapter 13).

- *Learning contract:* basically means the same as above. The word *contract* is more formal but, whether it is an 'agreement' or a 'contract' you make with your mentor, you must complete it, as agreed, if you want to be successful.

- *Learning objectives:* a term used to describe the specific things that the student will demonstrate by the end of the placement. The term is sometimes used interchangeably with the term *learning outcomes*.

- *Learning opportunities:* a term used to describe all the identified aspects of nursing that you are able to experience in a clinical placement. These may be formal and expected or informal and take place by chance.

- *Learning environments:* a term used to describe the setting where learning takes place. This can be as diverse as an outpatient clinic, an operating theatre, a social care home, a patient's own home and many more.

- *Learning diary:* a term used to describe your personal record of the experiences and learning that you experience from within each placement. You can record your thoughts as often as you like and the diary can take many forms.

- *Proficiencies:* a term used to describe the specific learning set by the NMC. Nursing programmes must provide the student with the opportunities to achieve the standard required. First-year student nurses must meet the '*outcomes* to be achieved for entry to the branch programme' (NMC 2004: 26).

- The *assessment of practice process* describes what you have to do in order to complete your assessment of practice, e.g. a formative and summative assessment with your mentor, achieve outcomes x, y and z, keep a practice journal, write a case study. More about this in Chapter 13.

- *Portfolio:* most universities require students to present all their evidence from practice in one place (more about this later). Rather than calling it a file or folder of evidence, it tends to be known as a portfolio.

- *Evidence:* takes many forms. It refers to the work that you produce for your portfolio, which confirms to the marker that you have achieved what you needed to (i.e. for the placement or for the practice module). It may be your mentor writing and signing a report about you, your learning outcomes signed off, etc.

+···

Exercise 9.1 Evidence

Skim read through the chapter now, spotting how many times the word evidence appears. Think about the different usage and what it tells you about gathering evidence when you are in practice.

···

9.3 **More about mentors**

In Chapter 2 we referred briefly to the role of the mentor, now we will say more. When student nurses are in clinical practice placements, the main responsibility for guiding their learning rests with an individual (nearly always a registered nurse) called a mentor. Your mentor is responsible for *supporting you, helping you to identify and meet your learning outcomes* and *assessing* your learning within the clinical environment.

Wherever you are studying, it is a requirement of your programme that you are supported by a mentor, whenever you are in practice. Your mentor knows from conversation with you, and with guidance from the university, what you need to learn when in the placement. It is the role of the mentor to ensure that you have access to the necessary *learning opportunities* in order to meet your *learning needs*. For this reason the student nurse–mentor relationship is the most important one you have in any placement.

Mentor comment

❝ I've been a mentor now in Accident and Emergency for 3 years. I qualified 5 years ago and after working on an orthopaedic ward for 6 months, I decided I really wanted to be here at the sharp end, and luckily enough, I managed to get a post here soon after that. I like having students with me, so Charge Nurse here suggested that I might like to be a Mentor and he enabled me to do the mentorship course. Being a mentor is great because it means I have to keep myself up-to-date to answer all the student's questions, and so it reinforces my own learning. ❞

Mentor comment

❝ I am a community learning disability nurse. I consider it a privilege to mentor students; to be able to contribute to their knowledge, experience and attitude development at the beginning of their career. As well as this, I aim to pass on my enthusiasm for this field of work. It is so satisfying to see students' abilities and confidence grow and watch them develop. ❞

Team mentorship

Busy environments sometimes take a team approach to mentorship. In practice this means you might learn alongside a variety of registered nurses during your placement. Some of the registered nurses will be mentors and others may be associate mentors or co-mentors. Check the terminology where you are placed. Whilst you might work alongside your mentor for the majority of your time in placement, there may be times where your mentor will be off-duty, or will be doing something else, and she will arrange for you to work with another member of the team, e.g. an associate mentor.

For every occasion you are in practice it is important to work under the overall guidance of a mentor. For example, if your mentor is unwell, you must take responsibility to ensure the nurse (or person) in charge allocates you a substitute mentor for the day/shift. Be patient and give the nurse in charge time to do this (e.g. at morning handover). However, if they do not realize that you are without a mentor (remember they have many more things to think about, as well as having a student nurse placed with them), gently remind them and wait to be told who this will be.

9.4 **Your mentor's role in your learning**

According to the NMC (2006), mentors:

1. **Organize and co-ordinate student learning activities in practice.**

   This does not mean that you cannot organize your own learning in addition to that which is organized by your mentor. In discussion with your mentor, you should actively seek new learning opportunities. However, your mentor will be familiar with the learning opportunities that are generally available within that particular setting.

2. **Supervise students in learning situations and provide them with constructive feedback on their achievements.**

   It is very important that you work alongside your mentor in clinical practice for the majority of the time. In some cases, and especially during this first year, your mentor may want to work very closely with you, in order to supervise what you are doing and to comment and feedback to you about your practice. Feedback is essential in helping you to identify when you have done something well; and will help you to repeat this practise in other, similar situations.

3. **Set and monitor realistic learning objectives for students.**

   Naturally when you enter clinical practice you want to see and learn everything you can. However, your learning needs should be realistic and pertinent to each clinical area. Your mentor can help you to refine your learning objectives to ensure that they are realistic and achievable. You also need to remember that your learning objectives may change as you progress through the course, so even if you return to the same placement later on in the programme, there will be new learning objectives to set and proficiencies to achieve.

4. **Assess the total performance of students, including their developing nursing skills, attitudes and behaviour.**

   Mentors are there to assess your clinical competence against the proficiencies laid down by the NMC; they are also there to monitor your professional behaviour. This means that your mentor is duty bound to discuss your professional behaviour with you (see Chapter 13 for more about assessment).

5. **Provide evidence, as required by programme providers (i.e. your university), of student achievement or lack of achievement.**

   Your mentor will meet regularly with you to discuss your progress and will document your progress. The mentor may highlight areas where you are doing well and are achieving your proficiencies and learning objectives, but the mentor should also tell you about areas where you need to develop and focus your efforts in order to pass all elements of the practice placement. These will also be documented.

6. **Liaise with nurse teachers to provide feedback, identify any concerns about the student's performance and agree action, as appropriate.**

   Mentors may discuss your progress with link teachers from the university. In some cases, the mentor may contact your personal teacher, as they know you best. If you are struggling in clinical practice (and this might be for a whole host of reasons: problems with transport, child care, ill health, etc.), then an action plan will be agreed between yourself, the mentor and your personal teacher or the link teacher, in order to support your development and help you to achieve your goals.

7. **Provide evidence of, or act as, a sign-off mentor with regards to making decisions about the achievement of proficiency.**

   Note that in your case as a year-one student, the above means achieving the outcomes to be achieved for entry to the branch programme (NMC 2004).

During the first year, almost everything is a new experience and so the list of learning opportunities is endless. Remember, you are not only thinking about what you need to learn, but also what you wish to learn. How you progress will, to some extent, depend upon what you have done in the past, how confident you are and what you want to learn. For example, for students completely new to the healthcare environment, learning opportunities can range from talking to patients right through to psychomotor nursing skills, such as giving injections.

Never underestimate the amount of learning opportunities there are on every placement. But if your learning is going to be effective, then you have to go into every placement with a positive attitude. Learning opportunities are everywhere, all the time—it is up to you to see them. Being curious, inquisitive, engaged and interested all help.

Student comment

66 Be *enthusiastic* (even if you have to fake it a bit sometimes) because if you don't look like, or say that, you want to learn and see things, then the staff and your mentor won't think of you when opportunities arise. Also, if you do miss opportunities, then talk to your mentor (be diplomatic of course) and ensure that next time you don't miss the opportunities. You really must push yourself out there, and not expect mentors to constantly spoon-feed you opportunities. 99

The mentor's role in your assessment

66 Your mentor is responsible for 'signing off' your documentation at the end of the placement to verify (confirm) that you have achieved your learning outcomes. For this reason students and mentors usually try to work at the same time and have the same days off to make working together as easy as possible. 99

Read more about this in Chapter 13.

9.5 How learning occurs in clinical practice placements

Exercise 9.2 Learning in practice

Learning occurs in many ways, as the following will show. Think about each section below as you read through and consider what you will do to maximize your learning in each of the ways described.

Observation

'Observation is to gather data by using the senses … [and] is a conscious, deliberate skill that is developed through effort' (Kozier *et al.* 2008: 148).

This is an essential skill for a registered nurse to use and is fundamental to your learning. As a first-year student, a good place to start is by observing your mentor. Your mentor is an experienced nurse (or non-nurse, as explained in Chapter 7) with lots of knowledge and expertise. As you work alongside your mentor, always *observe* what she or he does.

When observing patients and clients we use our senses. Observation involves:

- *Looking:* What can you see? Facial expression; do you see a smile or a grimace? Body language; is it comfortable or tense? Has the person eaten all their lunch or left most of it? Are they upset? Withdrawn, sitting alone? Are they cyanosed (with a blue tinge to the lips and nose)?

- *Hearing:* Listen to what is being said, the content of the speech. Notice sighs or yawning, silences or pressure of speech (that is when someone speaks very quickly) or the slurring of words. What do these things suggest to you?

- *Touch:* Clammy or hot skin can indicate raised temperature. A sudden change to a rapid pulse or very slow pulse can indicate ill health.

- *Smell:* Does the patient need help with personal hygiene? Can you smell alcohol? Is their breath malodorous?

However, observation on its own has limitations. Experienced nurses have an uncanny knack of being able to pass by the bottom of the patients' bed, or to have a conversation with a sick child or a person with learning disability and know that there is something not right about them. Skilled mental health nurses can ask one or two questions and seem to be able to instantly zero in on what the problem is and can then do something about it. Nurses who work with people with learning disability can sometimes *sense* they are not happy or comfortable. This ability is known as expertise.

Being inquisitive and curious

Observing your mentor is one thing, *questioning* why they practised in a certain way is another thing altogether.

+ ....

Exercise 9.3 Education or training?

Pause here for a moment and think about the difference between being *educated* to do something and being *trained*. You are on a programme of nurse education. What important message does this give you?

....

In 2010 it is not the intention of the NMC that you are *being trained* to be a nurse; animals are trained and are unthinking about what they have been trained to do, they just do it. You are not being trained just to copy your mentor, you are being *educated* to understand why your mentor is doing something and then to practice yourself with knowledge and confidence in your actions.

Much of your mentors' expert knowledge is carried in his or her head. It will be hidden from you unless you can find a way of teasing out that knowledge. It is these mental processes (how they are thinking, problem-solving, deciding what action to take, weighing up alternative nursing interventions, etc.) that you need to learn in order to develop your own expertise.

The challenge for you is that experts can often find it difficult to say how they know what they know; particularly whilst an action is taking place. So, observing someone is all well and good and might enable you to perform a certain task by repeating what you see, but this will only tell you *how* to do something. The real skill and knowledge comes from knowing *when and why* to do something, as well as how. The key to moving on from observation and being inquisitive is asking questions.

Asking questions

This might seem like a simple and obvious thing, but you have to keep asking questions of your mentor to understand the processes that they are going through, whenever they observe or talk to a patient or client. What are they thinking? Of course there are ways and means of asking questions and you should consider the impact of your questioning. Be careful to explain to your mentor that you are really keen to learn; you are not trying to be difficult.

Use your judgement (common sense) about questions that should *not* be asked in front of patients. Note this includes people who have learning disability, Alzheimer's disease, who are unconscious, terminally ill or just hard of hearing. It is impossible to know how much people can hear and understand in these cases. Also remember that curtains round beds are not sound-proofed! The physical barrier they provide prevents others *seeing* what is going on, but not *hearing*.

+ ···

Exercise 9.4 Open questions

Notice how, when you ask open questions, you get a better reply.

Please explain why you did that?

What would have been another way to approach the situation?

Why do you think X happened?

Now think of some of your own to vary your questioning.

···

Listening to, and learning from, patients, clients and their families

People know themselves best; so it follows that they are the best people to talk to about their *condition* (i.e. their mental or physical ill health). In some cases, the patient is the *only* person who can provide the kind of detailed information about what it is like to live with a certain condition, or have a family member who has that condition. Try to get used to talking to, and really listening to, what patients wish to share with you about their lives. As a student you are supernumerary and so may be one of the few people who can really spend time talking and listening to patients, clients and their families.

It might seem quite strange at first to initiate a conversation with someone who you don't know, but like anything else, it is easier with practice. You could start by asking if it is OK for you to spend a few minutes talking to them about what has brought them into hospital; ask them about how their problem has impacted on various aspects of their lives, roles and relationships within the family, attitudes to health and illness and so on. There are a multitude of things for you to find out, and all the information you can gather will ultimately help you to add to your personal *mental library* of experiences.

If you are going to talk to a patient, client or family, then make sure you remember to maintain their confidentiality; this might mean asking if they would talk to you somewhere more private or quieter than the middle of a busy ward. Try to find a quiet spot. Think about the environment, making sure that the room is a comfortable temperature, that you are not likely to be disturbed by people coming in and out, or a telephone ringing, and make sure that the person is comfortable before you start. It is also a good idea to sit at the same level as the other person. Talking to patients and clients at the same time as doing a dozen other things is not ideal. Give the person the attention they deserve (see Figure 9.1).

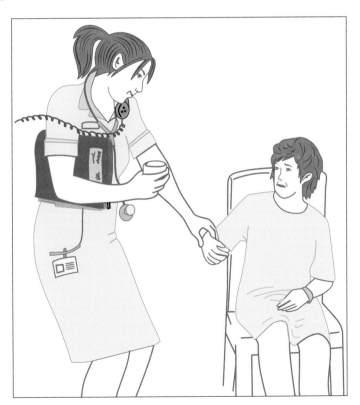

Figure 9.1 Nurse multi-tasking and not giving proper attention to the patient. Artist: Emma Heaton

Being proactive, using initiative

A *proactive* student nurse will actively be engaging in his or her learning and seeking out learning opportunities. Occasionally you may need to be proactive in organizing your mentor. Remember, your mentor is not only responsible for facilitating your learning, but also will have patients to nurse. At times you may need to be gently assertive (see Chapter 3) and take the lead in reminding him or her about the learning objectives that you want to achieve. Try to take some 'time out' each shift for a quick discussion about what you have learned that day, the milestones you have met or to go over things that you need some clarification on. You may also need to remind your mentor about how many weeks you have on the placement and when you need to have met all the objectives.

Participating

To learn well you need to participate in the total activity of the placement. Your activities will be determined by the needs of the patients, clients or children there. This may be 'hands on', e.g. helping patients to wash and dress; giving injections; or undertaking wound dressings. Alternatively it might be joining in an activity with a person with learning disability, such as accompanying them shopping or swimming, supporting them to eat and drink, or supervising as they do something themselves, such as boiling a kettle. A mental health placement in the community may involve visiting a patient at home with his family for the first time, observing the nurse assess the person's needs. Under supervision, a children's nursing student may bottle-feed an infant.

Mentor comment

❝ If you feel you have been asked to do something that is above your level of understanding or that you have not seen or experienced before, you should not participate until you feel comfortable to do so. Saying that you don't feel ready to take on a task, or have never seen it done before, might seem like a daunting prospect at first, but remember, everyone has to start somewhere. ❞

In practice your mentor, or another registered nurse, will demonstrate the activity and explain the underpinning theory first, then you observe the task in practice, then gradually you take on elements of the task and your mentor steps back, allowing you to develop and refine the skill. So you can see that it is really important to be able to talk to your mentor about what your previous experience is and what you are comfortable with. Of course, it is the job of your mentor to help you to develop your skills and, at times, this might mean really pushing you within that comfort zone. So it is a difficult balance for both of you.

A good relationship with your mentor is essential so that you can both get the most from each other and you can get the most from the placement. Gradually, your confidence will grow and your mentor will encourage you to do more and more, and then you can negotiate with your mentor when you feel ready to undertake the skill on your own, under his or her supervision. Observation is a great way to learn, but there comes a time when you must do it yourself.

The best way to get the most from your mentor is to make sure that you participate in all the activities that contribute to patient care. You might do this through observation, supported participation and eventually independently, but learning through *doing* is really effective. You may also need to be quite assertive in pushing yourself forward in order to make the most of all the learning opportunities. Indeed, you may have to be somewhat selfish to ensure that you are not forgotten about when there is something interesting for you to observe or participate in.

Learning from a mentor talking through her actions

Ask your mentor to talk you through what they are doing and to verbally guide you as you undertake the task. If the mentor is able to tell you about the kinds of thoughts she is having related to the activity, or the kinds of questions she is asking herself, you can use similar sets of thoughts and questions yourself to improve your own problem-solving skills. Gradually, you will build up your own mental library of experiences and situations, and you will remember sets of thoughts and questions that are associated with particular patient or client needs. This helps you to develop your own expertise. You can mentally sift through the irrelevant thoughts and questions, and begin to zero in on what is relevant and important. What you are doing here is learning to recognize patterns of needs, problems, signs and symptoms, and match them to your previous experiences. The impact of this on your learning should not be underestimated. So working together, talking together and thinking aloud together are really useful mechanisms to boost your learning.

• • • **A word about** Thinking out loud

It is not always wise to do this in front of the patient or client, so you might need to combine observation first with discussion afterwards. In different circumstances, where a person is actively engaged in their own care, this might be different. Always be guided by your mentor.

Learning by identifying and pursuing your own learning goals/objectives

At first you might be a little overwhelmed by the placement. There can be a lot of fast-paced activity in acute care settings, be they in a mental health, child or adult placement. If you are unfamiliar with people with learning disability, it can take a while to get to know them and settle. Identifying some *personal learning goals* (i.e. things you would like specifically to learn/experience in the placement) will help you to focus on one or two activities at first, and stop you feeling overwhelmed by trying to make sense of everything that is going on.

Mentor comment

" If you struggle to identify learning goals of your own, through which to achieve the outcomes, then do not worry. Many placements will have identified certain practice-based learning activities that are open for first-year students. "

As explained above, learning opportunities exist in almost every single patient or client encounter in *all* your placements. The following example shows the learning available in something that you might (at this point) see as a basic nursing task, not a nursing skill at all: helping someone to wash and dress.

! Fact box Learning opportunity example

The skin is the largest organ of the body. A nurse needs knowledge of the structure and function of the skin (anatomy and physiology) to be able to relate the observations to the physiology. Helping someone to wash enables you to observe and monitor the condition of the skin. If the skin is dry and flaky, the person may be dehydrated and not taking in enough fluid; if the skin is hot, the patient may have a raised temperature caused by an infection; if the skin is clammy, the patient may be in pain; if the skin is mottled and slightly blue in appearance, then the patient may not be getting enough oxygenated blood around the body. This list could go on!

So you can see that simply by observing the skin, this can lead a registered nurse to a range of questions or thoughts about what is going on physiologically within the patient. This may in turn lead the nurse to try and resolve the patient's problem.

Keeping a learning diary

Your experiences in clinical practice are extremely important in learning to be a nurse and there are many ways in which you can use your experiences in order to help you to learn; keeping a learning diary is one of those. A learning diary is a personal record, which you can keep private or you may choose to use aspects from your diary in discussions with your mentor or personal teacher. A learning diary is also a handy way of remembering what you did in each placement and will provide you with a record of your development throughout the course (see Figure 9.2). There are no hard and fast rules about keeping a learning diary; the style, form and content will be personal to you. You might want to write something

Monday 17th January

My first call this morning was to get a lady off the commode. She told me she had done her sample so I took the opportunity to do a urinalysis which showed up an increase in leukocytes. When I went to write the result in the doctors' book I realized that it had already been reported.

Learning: Check doctors' book first next time. Also, not to be too hard on myself for the repetition of this; I was using my initiative to do something I know I could do, and trying to be helpful.

After that I changed and made beds. I started off wearing gloves and an apron, but soon got rid of the gloves and opted for hand rub in between doing each bed.

Learning: Tonight I have read that hand rub does not kill noroviruses, nor does it kill bacteria I spores - so I am not sure of its point? Should I just wash my hands between beds? I must ask the infection control nurse about this as I know there is a real risk of patient to patient contamination through me when bed making.

Then I helped washing and dressing in the men's bay. I used the standing hoist again. I find it so cumbersome and time-consuming, and there is a lot of bending around to make sure the patient's feet are where they should be? Plus you need two people to use it and it is a part for infection.

Learning: Sometimes nursing can be a frustrating activity! But it is necessary to save our backs and for health and safety. So I just better learn to love that hoist!

Figure 9.2 Example of a student learning diary entry

at the end of each shift or every week; you might want a traditional paper-based document or use a voice recorder . . . the options are endless.

Visits

Whilst you are allocated to a particular placement there will often be opportunities for you to make visits to associated areas of the health and social care services. For example, an outpatient's clinic, community resource, walk-in centre, or drug and alcohol team.

You may know people who work within health and social care who volunteer to take you with them for experience. They may work within your usual Trust, but may not. Remember that all learning placements have to be audited and passed as suitable learning environments and so you should make absolutely sure that your university supports this kind of activity before you go.

In an adult or child placement, you might like to think about ensuring that you follow the patient journey from admission to discharge. Perhaps you could talk to your mentor about ensuring that you care for the same group of patients during your time on the ward. You might be able to organize accompanying the patient (with additional supervision) to other departments, such as X-ray or theatre. This will help you to make sense of the patient experience and appreciate what the patient goes through. In a learning disability setting, try to ensure you spend sometime with the clients in a range of venues, not just where they live or spend the day. The list of potential learning opportunities is endless and Chapter 11 will also give you more ideas.

Learning from your peer group in practice

You will be surrounded by fellow students throughout this first year of your course. Initially you will feel like newcomers but not for long. Your fellow students are a valuable resource for friendship, support and knowledge. Although common foundation students are working towards the same learning outcomes, some of your colleagues may have different clinical placements and experiences. So you might find it beneficial to talk to them about those experiences, in order for you to begin to establish in your mind what the differences and similarities are between the different branches of nursing.

Many students talk about developing enduring friendships with their fellow students, which helps them to get through the demanding world of clinical practice (Roberts 2007). It is important to remember that every one of you will have your own unique experiences, but many of your peers will have experienced very similar situations to yourself. You could also talk to students who are slightly further on in the course than yourself. These students are often able to offer valuable advice and insider knowledge about getting through your clinical placements. However, just because a fellow student did not enjoy a particular placement, this does not necessarily mean that you will have a similar experience.

Learning from complaints

Patients, clients and their families may wish to make complaints about any aspect of their encounters with the health service and you will need to be aware of the local procedures for dealing with such complaints. You should never ignore a complaint but remember that you may not be the right person to deal with the complaint, since you are not accountable and responsible in the same way that a qualified nurse is. Read more about learning from complaints in Chapter 14.

+···

Exercise 9.5

Visit the Parliamentary and Health Service Ombudsman website and see what kinds of complaints might be made.
http://www.ombudsman.org.uk/improving_services/special_reports/hsc/nhs_remedy/ index.html

···

How to learn from something you have done that was not correct

It is unlikely that you will complete your programme without (at some time) doing something incorrectly. The important thing is to learn from your error and not to repeat your mistake. Sometimes a mistake or incorrect practise can have consequences for the patient, client or their family. If you think you may have made a mistake you *must* tell your mentor, no matter how difficult this might seem. Your mentor can discuss the situation with you and support you through whatever happens following the discussion.

You might also need to go and speak to the patient, client or their family in person, explaining what happened and, of course, you should apologize for your actions and state clearly how the situation will be remedied. You may also need to record the incident in the patient's nursing notes.

+ ....

Exercise 9.6 Apologizing

If you ever need to apologize the following may help:

- Take responsibility for what happened.
- Explain how it happened.
- Show how it won't happen again.
- Apologize in a way that shows you mean it, be sincere.

....

Working with your mentor

In an ideal world you would always learn *alongside* your mentor or a registered nurse. However, for various reasons, this is not always possible. Examples of circumstances that could get in the way of this are as follows:

- In an emergency situation, your mentor will prioritize the situation over your learning.
- Where there are staff shortages, your mentor must go where they are needed to support patient and client care. You may not always be able to join them there.
- If a patient declines to have you as a student working with them, a patient's or client's wish for privacy outweighs your desire for interesting learning opportunities, *with no exception*.

What does the content above tell you about the student nurse–mentor relationship?

That it is important that you understand that being '*guided by your mentor*' does not always mean you must be 'joined at the hip' in close proximity to each other while you are caring for patients. This occasional distance does not alter the fact that when in practice as a first-year student you are *always* under direct supervision.

9.6 **Mentors and learning in non-NHS settings**

• • • **A word about** Non-nurse mentors

As we explained in Chapter 7, in certain areas for *some* of your practice experiences in the first year, you *may* go to non-NHS placements. For example, a learning disability social care home run by the local authority or to a service run by Scope (a voluntary sector service with residential settings in some areas). For a child health experience, you may go to a local nursery or even a school. In these placements you will rarely have a nurse as your mentor, but you will have a suitably qualified and experienced person in their own field (social care work, education, etc.) to assess your practice in their placement.

Even in a non-NHS placement:

- The placement has been audited by nurse teachers as a learning environment.
- Your mentor has been given guidance from the university as to how to perform this role.
- There is a link teacher from the university who is responsible for the placement (the role of the link or liaison teacher was introduced in Chapter 2).

It is possible to learn a great deal of useful things in these non-NHS placements and the experience can help you appreciate how care is delivered in other settings.

9.7 **How you may work with your mentor in practice**

If you have been working with your mentor for a few days and have discussed your previous experience of providing personal care in earlier placements, it would be quite acceptable for you to help a patient to get washed and dressed, whilst your mentor nurses another patient. On a mental health unit, if you have been guided by your mentor on how to observe a patient who is unwell, and you know how to identify the risks to the person and how to summon help if needed, it is acceptable that for a short time you take responsibility to observe the person, but only if you feel confident to do so.

Supervision and accountability

As a first-year student nurse, everything you do in practice is under the supervision of a registered nurse mentor who is accountable to the profession for your actions. You must understand that their accountability to the profession for your actions *does not alter the fact that you also take full responsibility for what you do all the time when in practice.* (See more about accountability in Chapter 14.)

What if you arrive in practice and your mentor is not there?

If the absence of your mentor is not raised with you by the nurse in charge (e.g. at handover), remind them that your mentor is away and ask who should supervise you that day. You should do this to ensure you practice safely under supervision. To be proactive, if you discover that next Thursday, when you are due to be in placement, your mentor will be on a study day, then you need to ensure another registered nurse has been named to mentor you for the day.

Communicating with your mentor

You must clarify with your mentor how you will communicate with each other throughout the placement. For example, agree how often you will have formal discussions about your progress and also how your informal communication will take place. You might want to discuss whether you are the sort of person who will ask lots of questions, or the sort of person who likes a lot of direction, or if you have any particular concerns about the placement.

Student comment

66 *Make friends with the care assistants and newly qualified nurses, they are useful resources. If there is a problem, don't stew, get on to your link tutor or mentor straight away. Try and get as much of the portfolio as you can do whilst in practice (especially signatures) because they will have forgotten you 10 minutes after you leave the ward.* 99

Summary

This chapter has introduced you to the role and functions of mentors in clinical practice and given you some ideas about what working with your mentor might be like. It has also outlined some of the many ways you learn in practice. There may be specifics that are unique to your university, but most of the common aspects have been included here. This chapter gives you a starting point, but of course it is now down to you to go into your clinical area with enthusiasm for learning. Remember, all opportunities are potential learning opportunities, but you need to grasp every one.

■ Top tips

- There will *never* be a placement where you cannot learn something.
- Whether or not you can *see the learning* is down to you.
- If you ring your personal tutor from a placement and say 'There is nothing to learn here', they will never agree with you!
- Understand that you will be learning about yourself as much as you are learning new skills.
- Appreciate all the different ways you can learn and use them.
- Enjoy and value your learning; you are entering a profession where your learning will never stop.

■ Online resource centre

To find links to websites where you can find more information on communication skills, dealing with complaints and the International Council of Nursing's advice on medication errors, go to: **www.oxfordtextbooks.co.uk/orc/hart/**

■ References

Kozier B, Erb G, Berman A, Snyder S, Lake R and Harvey S (2008) *Fundamentals of nursing: Concepts, process and practice*. Pearson Education, Harlow, England.

Roberts D (2007) Friendships and the community of students: peer learning amongst a group of pre-registration student nurses. Unpublished PhD thesis, The University of Salford.

NMC (2004) *Standards of proficiency for pre-registration nursing education*. Standards 02 04. NMC, London.

NMC (2006) *Standards to support learning and assessment in practice NMC standards for mentors, practice teachers and teachers*. Standards 08 06. NMC, London.

First steps into practice

Debbie Roberts

The aims of this chapter are:

➤ To help you feel confident to enter your placement for the first time

➤ To provide practical advice

➤ To introduce you to some of the people you will meet

This chapter is full of practical tips to help your first steps into practice. Whether or not you have had previous experience of working in healthcare settings, this is likely to be a challenging experience for you. Rather like your first day at university, you will be meeting new people, in an unfamiliar environment. You will have to meet your mentor, the nurse (or other person) in charge of the placement and the staff team for the first time. From the outset there will be certain expectations of you as a student nurse, e.g. it will be assumed that you are there because you want to learn and that you will conduct yourself in a manner fitting a future registered nurse (more about this in Chapters 14 and 15).

10.1 Before your first placement

If you have:

* read Chapters 7, 8 and 9 of this book;

* attended all the preparation sessions at uni;

* read through the paperwork you have been given; and

* called in or telephoned the placement in advance; and

* found out as much as you can about the placement; and

* know exactly who you are meeting at what time and where . . .

. . . then you have done a great deal to prepare yourself and you will be feeling a lot more confident than your colleagues who have not done these things! Some pre-placement nerves are normal. So do not worry. Build your confidence now by reading on, making sure you apply all the issues covered here to your own circumstances. The topics covered are equally applicable to placements everywhere: community, hospital, residential service, school and nursery.

Student comment

66 Make sure you organize child care, if required. Remember student nurses have to work 'earlies' (early shifts), 'lates' and weekends. 99

Pack a bag

It helps to know what to take with you and what to leave at home on your first day.

Paperwork

You will need to take your paperwork for the assessment of your practice. The assessment will *not* start on your first day, but will be needed later. The paperwork will include a form that will need to be filled in on your first or second day called 'orientation to placement' (or something similar). See Chapter 13 for more about assessment in practice.

Your paperwork is your responsibility. Keep it in a safe place whilst in practice so that it does not become lost or spoiled. Take it home with you at the end of each shift.

• • • **A word about** Paperwork and your mentor

It is *not a good idea* to let your mentor take your practice documents home for completion because:

- As Chapter 13 will explain, they are not doing the assessment *on you* they are doing it *with you*; you should be there for all discussions to confirm how you met the outcomes.
- What if they have taken your portfolio, then they have a family emergency, and are not at work for 3 weeks. Explain that back at uni!

Notebook and pen

Student comment

66 It is a good idea to carry a small notebook and jot down information as you go along; it's surprising what you forget and how quickly. However, remember, if some of what you are noting down is *confidential information*, make sure nobody but you see it and that it is destroyed at the end of the shift (remove and shred the pages). 99

If you have a pocket-sized notebook and pen with you, if you come across words or phrases that you do not understand, jot them down to look up later. If you are not in an area where name badges are worn (e.g. a learning disability day service), you can also easily jot down the names of staff to remind yourself who they are.

In an adult setting, if you are given a series of tasks to perform (e.g. urinalysis for Mr X, blood pressure check for Mrs Y, check catheter bag for Ms P and check fluid chart of Mrs H), a quick look back at your notes will ensure that Mrs Y is not surprised when you ask her for a urine sample and Ms P is not unduly worried that her blood pressure may be a cause for concern.

Student comment

" Carry an address or notebook with alphabetical pages. When you come across a drug you are not familiar with, write it down to look up later. "

Student comment

" Get a torch, as you will need one at some point, even if not in the first year, certainly before you go on night duty. On a hospital ward, trying to check catheters in the middle of the night using the light from your car key fob is quite difficult, and the patient wonders what you are doing crawling under their bed! "

Money and valuables

Unless you know there are secure facilities (such as a locker) available in your placement, it makes sense to take just enough money for coffee and lunch, and to leave valuables at home. This advice is particularly true if your placement is in a hospital. Hospitals are public places and, as such, are always vulnerable to opportunist thefts.

Food/snacks

This may not be necessary if your placement is in a hospital with a staff café, but if you are placed anywhere remote (e.g. a residential setting in a rural area), then you may be glad you put a sandwich or a cereal bar and apple in your bag. From your second day on you will know whether food is available. If you are going to be out with a community nurse, take a bottle of water too (better than a can of drink because you can take sips all day).

Student comment

❝ Take plenty of food that's easy to eat in small bites, as sometimes you don't get a break. If you are offered a break, take it. No one will thank you for not doing so. ❞

A watch

From day one you need to have immediate access to find out the exact time whenever you need know it. *Do not rely* on clocks, other people or using your mobile 'phone for this purpose. Why? Your mobile 'phone must be switched off when you are in your placement and be locked away safely (see Chapter 14). Clocks are seldom in the right place when you need one, and in any case may be inaccurate or have stopped. Other people may be too busy to want to be disturbed by you asking the time.

A watch will help you to arrive on time, meet your mentor at the time you agreed (not five minutes early or late) and when you say to a patient or client (as doubtless you will have the need to sometime) 'I will pop back and see how you are in x minutes' that you keep your promise. A watch will prevent a 30-minute break from stretching into 40 minutes (and the concern about your lack of professionalism that such behaviour would convey to your mentor).

When in practice, a watch will also help you work out *how long* you have for certain activities. For example, in a residential service for people with learning disability, your mentor suggests you spend the next hour reading through the person-centred care plans for *all* the five residents, to help you get a *feel* for how the staff team work with them. You need to spend about 12 minutes looking at each one to achieve this. Spending 30 minutes reading about resident one will mean you will have to skim read through the others, and you will not be doing as you have been asked. (Go back to Chapter 4 if you are still struggling with time-management.)

A watch with a second hand is useful, particularly for recording physiological observations. For example, you will need to feel a patients' pulse and count the beats for a full minute. Depending on where you are working, you may need to keep your watch pinned inside your pocket. Remember to check the uniform policy.

Self-presentation

It goes without saying that your personal hygiene should be exemplary: clean skin and hair, and fresh breath. Before your placement starts, remove nail varnish and piercings (if necessary) and think about what you will do with your hair if it is long. Have a soak in the bath now and ease your pre-placement jitters, or else set your alarm for enough time for a shower in the morning. In the morning, remember no perfume or after shave with a strong aroma. Both can induce feelings of nausea in patients. Read Chapter 14 for more about appearance.

Organize your clothes

You will have been advised about what the uniform consists of (e.g. tunic and trousers), so get it ready exactly as it should be worn. As you know by now, regardless of your future branch of nursing you will be on your feet for long periods, so remember to wear comfortable shoes. On your first day, and every day afterwards, your uniform should be freshly laundered and ironed. If you are wearing a uniform you must attach your name badge.

> **Mentor comment**
>
> 66 Some hospitals will offer facilities to launder your uniform for you. Be sure to find this out. 99

Remember some placements will allow you to wear a wedding ring, but this is usually the only form of jewellery allowed. Sikh students may be permitted to wear the Kara and female Muslim students can continue to wear the Hijab, but there may be restrictions about what colour it should be and you need to check this out.

! Fact box

Hijab: a scarf worn by female Muslims, which covers the head and hair. Usually a veil is not worn by nursing students; the face is left exposed.

Kara: a bangle worn by both male and female Sikhs. This is a sacred piece of jewellery and must not be removed.

See Holland and Hogg (2001) in the further reading list.

Your appearance is of utmost importance. Patients need to feel that they are going to be well looked after by you, and so you need to project an air of quiet confidence. When people feel ill and vulnerable, you need to make them feel safe and cared for, and your uniform is an important aspect of creating a positive image of nurses and nursing.

Non-uniform (mufti) placements

In some areas it is customary for nurses not to wear uniform, but instead normal, everyday clothes. This is particularly true in less clinical environments, such as mental health and learning disability placements. However, there is likely to be a dress code that you need to be aware of and adhere to in these placements. The rules about jewellery might still apply, so once again, you will need to check this out before you start your first shift. Some placements might consider jeans and a T-shirt to be fine, but other areas might not. You need to remember that you are a student nurse developing a professional role, and are learning and working, so your usual dress outside of work, might not be the same thing as 'work wear'. See Chapter 14 for more advice.

Nurse teacher comment

❝ Always carry your university ID and name badge with you to placements. You never know when you may be asked to confirm who you are. ❞

What time are you due to start?

Student comment

❝ Working shifts for the first time really upset my system. I could not sleep properly and could not work out when to eat. Within a few months I had put on a lot of weight. My uniform was not fitting. I knew I had to do something about it—but then went much too far the other way and lost loads of the weight I had put on and more. People thought I was ill. I was not ill—I was just thrown into a pattern that did not naturally suit me and it took a lot of working out for me. I am OK now. ❞

If you are not used to getting up at 05.30 or 06.00 to go to work, you will have to be confident that your alarm will not let you down (using two, a clock *and* your mobile may help here). You may sleep restlessly (after all tomorrow is a big day). Thinking of this as *excitement* and *anticipation* is more positive than thinking of it as nerves.

The exact times you will be required to be in your placement may vary according to whether you are a full-time or part-time (extended programme) student, and the standard working hours for the regular (established) staff in the area where you have been allocated for your clinical practice. As a rule of thumb, when in practice it is usual for pre-registration student nurses who are doing a full-time programme to follow the standard working hours that the regular full-time staff observe. This is so you are there for the key events (such as handovers) and in the placement for as much time as your mentor.

Shift work start times vary, but in any placement where the clients have been sleeping the night (hospital, residential service, assessment and treatment unit) they will start early, say between seven and eight o'clock in the morning. A shift would typically be until between 15.00 and 16.30. The afternoon or 'late shift' would usually start at around lunchtime and you would work until around 21.00.

Mon	Tues	Wed	Thurs	Fri	Sat	Sun	Mon	Tues	Wed	Thurs	Fri	Sat	Sun
L	off	L	off	E	E	L	E	L	E	L	E	off	off

Table 10.1 Extract from an 'off duty' rota.

> **! Fact box** A 'day' shift explained
>
> In care settings where shift work is the norm, nurses generally work 'earlies', 'lates' or nights. If in such an area a person does a 'day', it means starting later than an early shift, and leaving before the late shift has ended (e.g. to work 9–5). To work like that covers both the 'early' and 'late' teams in the area, so is good for communication. However, working such times means missing the handovers and never seeing the night staff, so these are negatives.

Students are expected to work a mixture of 'earlies' (E) and 'lates' (L) each week and to have 2 days off (but these may not be together). Two weeks 'off-duty' might look something like Table 10.1.

Normally student nurses are not expected to work Bank Holidays whilst in clinical practice, but this may not be the case where you are studying. In the UK most Bank Holidays fall around Christian festivals, so if you are of a different faith, you should speak to your personal teacher or mentor about having time off when it is more fitting for you. For example, if you are a Muslim student, you may prefer to work at Christmas but take time off to celebrate Eid.

During your pre-registration programme there is a requirement for you to experience the full 24-hour cycle of care, including night duty. However, many universities and/or clinical areas prefer students not to undertake night duty during the first 6 months or even later in the programme. You will be expected to work some weekends.

> **? Stop and think**
>
> If you have never worked in a job that requires you to do shifts before, the 'off-duty' (Table 10.1) may look challenging. It will help you to be ready for your placements if you start to consider the impact shift work may have on your current living circumstances now. Are you going to be able to play football on Saturday and train in mid-week? What about the school run? If you are new to shift work it can take some time to get used to. Chapter 4 offers some helpful hints about managing your time.

How are you going to get there?

Student comment

66 Do not be late. Make sure you 'suss' out parking and how long it will take you to get there, as first impressions do count and you do not want to be flustered on your first day!. 99

Work out your journey, be it train, bus, car or walk. Factor in enough time for some delay. If you are driving, know where you are going to park. See Chapter 8 for further guidance.

Punctuality

You should *never* arrive late on duty without telephoning ahead to let them know, and always offer to make up the time at the end of the shift or on another occasion. This might seem pedantic, but the NMC requires you to complete a certain number of hours in clinical practice, and so every hour has to be accounted for. If you are sick or absent, then you will be advised by your nurse teachers if, and how much, practice time you will have to make up before the end of the course. So it's really important that you try and take good care of yourself, keeping yourself fit and healthy (see Chapter 3).

Student comment

66 Make sure you can get to your placement for a 7 a.m. start, or can get home late at night, especially if you are relying on public transport. Do a dummy run, if necessary, at those times. 99

10.2 **On arrival**

It is your first day and a big event for you, but for the regular staff, and a lot of the clients and patients, it is just another day. Be realistic; accept you are another of many student nurses who have passed their way. Try not to be too disappointed that they have not put the flags out to signal your arrival because they will not have. Thank all who take the time to welcome you. If they do not do so, recognize this for what it is: busy professionals with a zillion other things on their minds and a lot of responsibility and people to care for. It is not intended as an insult.

Meeting your mentor

You have the right to expect more of a welcome from your mentor. They are expecting you, especially if you called in advance, and want to work well with you. Listen carefully and follow to the letter all their instructions for the day.

What will you do?

Although you may hope to hit the ground running, with an interesting case conference, a couple of excellent nursing interventions or procedures to observe and an emergency for good measure, do not be disappointed. The reality is you may not see or do a lot on your first day. It takes time to settle in and most certainly in a learning disability and mental health placement, understanding more about the clients (through reading care plans) is necessary. Likewise you cannot expect to start working with children and their families from day one. Observe, listen and remember the messages in Chapter 9 about how you learn.

Orientation

To be *orientated* simply means that you have been shown around the placement, and helped to become familiar with the environment. There will be an orientation form for each placement (or something with a similar name in your portfolio), which is a useful guide to find out all the essential things you need to know, e.g. where are the fire alarms, fire extinguishers and emergency exits? If the placement gives you a new student information pack, read it.

Handover

This may be the first big *event* for you. Communication is very important, and nurses and other members of the team pass on important information to each other at the start of the shift in the form of a report. You will hear about how the clients and patients have been in the last hours and the work priorities for the new shift. Will there be a case conference, consultant round, theatre list, discharges, outings or any number of different events happening in your first day? Listen and observe.

10.3 **How to behave**

Wherever you are, you are a newcomer and a guest. Take an interest in everybody and everything going on. Remember, the message your body language gives is just as important as anything you say. Remember professional behaviour.

If there is a malodorous smell or something you are not used to (e.g. an incontinent patient has soiled their nightgown and sheets and is having a bed bath), remember the patient's feelings. A grimace will only make matters worse.

If a patient or relative speaks to you, say are a new student nurse and that you cannot help at the moment; then immediately seek advice from another team member.

Keep questions and queries for when your mentor has a spare moment; do not interrupt her when she is talking to someone else, unless it is urgent. Be patient, jot down your question and ask it later.

Answering the placement telephone, taking messages and using the computer

Check with your mentor the ground rules in your placement regarding these activities.

If you are permitted to answer the 'phone, do so by saying the location and then your designation (student nurse), followed by your first and last name. Then ask who is speaking and offer to help. Focus on the call and not on whatever task you were doing previously; this will distract you from what the caller is saying. Speak clearly and not too quickly. Tell the caller what you are going to do before you do it, e.g. 'I am going to put you on hold, find staff nurse Patel and say you wish to speak to her'. This sentence will give the caller confidence that you understood, and present you as helpful in meeting their request. Run the necessary errand immediately (no do not get distracted and forget!). Return to the caller if staff nurse is unavailable, offer further help or take a message. Above all be helpful and courteous. Thank them for calling, say goodbye. See this as professional behaviour development.

Always use the placement vehicle for message-taking (often a message book) and not the back of an envelope or scrap paper. Time and date the message, and say who it is for. Write clearly and ask the caller to spell any unfamiliar words.

If you are permitted to use the computer, do so only for issues related to your placement or your programme, and nothing else.

10.4 What to do in an emergency

This varies according to the client group you are working with and where you are placed. In a residential care home, an emergency may require a 999 call for police, fire or ambulance. In a hospital for medical emergencies, at least help is closer to hand.

If you find a patient in a collapsed state and you suspect that they are not breathing or their heart has stopped beating, you should call for help and pull the emergency bell (these are usually red in most areas). All hospitals and many care homes have these.

Don't worry if the patient has fainted, or is even just in a deep sleep, you must call for help first and then if the patient wakes up with all the commotion, you can tell them that you made a mistake. Never worry about using the emergency buzzer or calling for help, that is what it is there for.

You will have been taught basic life support in university and can commence the procedure according to what you have been taught and step back once more senior help arrives. But if you find the collapsed person, do not wait for others to arrive:

- ensure a safe approach;
- shout and shake;
- assess airway, breathing and circulation (ABC);
- commence CPR (cardiopulmonary resuscitation).

For further information check the following website on a regular basis for the most up-to-date resuscitation advice: **http://www.resus.org.uk/siteindx.htm**.

In a hospital, if you hear the emergency bell ringing, it usually means that a patient is in a life-threatening situation and help is required immediately to restore breathing and circulation. You will often see a flashing red light near to where the bell has been used, to tell you where the incident is. You may be required to take the emergency equipment to the scene. The equipment is usually kept together and is often referred to as the 'crash trolley', but there may be separate equipment, such as oxygen cylinders and suction machines, which may also need to be taken to the scene. You may be able to observe what is going on, or you might participate. The action will be fast-paced and you might feel surprisingly calm at the time, indeed it might feel a bit like everything is happening in slow motion around you. If you are able to take a step back and observe what is going on, try to look at what each member of the team is doing and how the team works together. Someone will be looking after the patient's airway and breathing, another will be undertaking chest compressions to maintain circulation and there is usually someone preparing drugs, which are often administered in sequences.

If you are not involved in the emergency situation (and remember that there is restricted room around a bedside, so don't be offended if you are asked to leave), try to ensure that other patients are supported. They may suspect what is happening and become quite concerned and anxious. There may also be family members who will need support. In some placements like Accident and Emergency, a member of staff might be specifically allocated to take care of the patients' relatives, so you might want to try and observe how they provide support at such difficult times.

The emergency situation may last for a few minutes or longer, depending on the situation and can result in both positive and negative outcomes. The patient may survive and need to be transferred to another ward or unit, or the resuscitation attempt may fail resulting in the death of the patient. In either case, you should take some time out to discuss the episode and your involvement in it with your mentor or personal teacher. You might want to try and write about what you observed and the feelings you encountered in your learning diary. An emergency situation can leave nurses (and students) feeling very emotional, whatever the outcome. Try to ensure that you talk about your feelings with your fellow students, mentor or teacher.

Epilepsy occurs more frequently in people with severe learning disability than in the rest of the population (NICE 2004). There are various types of seizures. To learn more, see the link to the NICE guidelines at the online resource. At first, seeing a seizure can be quite shocking, but in fact often a person recovers within a short space of time. Your mentor will recognize the circumstances where a seizure is more serious, such as in a condition known as status epilepticus, and observe how they respond.

10.5 Settling in to the placement

During each shift you will usually have a short break for a quick drink, of about 15–20 minutes and longer lunch break, between 30 minutes and 1 hour, so you can have something to eat.

Mentor comment

66 Working on placement requires energy, so make sure you have breakfast, remember to eat something at break time and lunch. You will not be able to function otherwise. If you are someone who 'never eats breakfast', it is time to change your ways! 99

Student comment

66 Always take your tea break when it is offered, as things change and develop so quickly you might not get one later. 99

What to do if you cannot attend your placement

Remember that if, for any reason, you cannot attend your placement, you should telephone and let them know. You should also let your personal teacher or someone at the university know that you have missed some time on clinical placement. There is usually a standard policy for reporting sickness and absence when you are in both university or out on placement, so make sure that you are aware of what the arrangements are. If you are unwell and cannot go in to work, then you can self-certify any sickness up to the first 7 days, after which you will need to submit a medical certificate, from your general practitioner (GP). Remember also to let both the clinical area and the university know, when you are well enough to return to work.

Student comment

❝ Get the healthcare assistants 'on your side'. Ask them to show you how to perform a task well, such as how to make a bed properly. They can make all the difference to a placement. If they like you, then your stay will be a lot more pleasant! Also, show that you are not afraid to 'muck in' and help–its amazing how much you can learn by doing this. ❞

Mentor comment

❝ Sometimes clients do not wish to have a student present and you must respect their wishes. ❞

See Chapter 14 for more information about this.

10.6 **Multi-disciplinary team members**

You know from Chapter 7 that nurses do not work in isolation and the multi-disciplinary team is the term used to describe the different professionals and other paid staff who work in health and social settings. The following gives a general overview of the roles. In Chapter 11 we will outline some of the specialist roles these individuals perform.

Physiotherapist

Physiotherapy sees movement as central to the health and well-being of individuals. They treat people of all ages with physical problems caused by illness, accident or ageing. For instance, they help people to regain function following surgery (such as a hip replacement) or following a stroke. Physiotherapists also help patients with breathing exercises and the clearing of secretions.
http://www.nhscareers.nhs.uk/details/Default.aspx?Id=281

Occupational therapist

Occupational therapy is the assessment and treatment of physical and psychiatric conditions using specific, purposeful activity to prevent disability and promote independent function in all aspects of daily life. An occupational therapist (OT) may give advice about aids and

adaptations that might help a person following a stroke, e.g. grab rails in the bathroom, easy grip handles on cutlery. OTs work in both hospital and community settings.
http://www.nhscareers.nhs.uk/details/Default.aspx?Id=281

Speech and language therapist

The role of a speech and language therapist (SALT) is to assess and treat speech, language and communication problems in people of all ages, to enable them to communicate to the best of their ability. They may also work with people who have eating and swallowing problems. Speech and language therapists work closely with teachers and health professionals. They use specialized skills to work directly with the client and provide support to them and their carers.
http://www.nhscareers.nhs.uk/details/Default.aspx?Id=281

Social worker

Social workers (case managers) form relationships with people and assist them to live more successfully in their local communities by helping them find solutions to their needs. Social workers engage not only with clients themselves but, if needed, their families and friends. They work closely with other organizations including the police, schools and the probation service.

Phlebotomist

Phlebotomists are specialized clinical support workers or assistant healthcare scientists who collect blood from patients for examination in laboratories, the results of which provide valuable information to diagnosing illness.
http://www.nhscareers.nhs.uk/details/Default.aspx?Id=281

Pharmacist

A pharmacist is an expert in medicines and their use. The majority of pharmacists practice in hospital pharmacy, community pharmacy or in primary care pharmacy. They provide information to patients on how to manage their medicines to ensure optimal treatment.
http://www.nhscareers.nhs.uk/details/Default.aspx?Id=281

Radiographer

There are two types of radiography: diagnostic and therapeutic. Diagnostic radiography uses a number of methods including X-rays to see if someone has broken a bone following a fall; whereas, therapeutic radiotherapy might be offered to a patient following the removal of a cancerous breast lump.
http://www.nhscareers.nhs.uk/details/Default.aspx?Id=189

··· **A word about** Nurse consultant roles

Nurse consultants are very experienced registered nurses, who will specialize in a particular field of healthcare. Each consultant role will be very different, depending upon the needs of the employer. Whatever the role, they are central to the process of health service modernization. All nurse consultants spend a minimum of 50% of their time working directly with patients, ensuring that people using the NHS continue to benefit from the very best nursing skills. In addition, the nurse consultants are responsible for developing personal practice, being involved in research and evaluation, and contributing to education, training and development.
http://www.nhscareers.nhs.uk/details/Default.aspx?Id=281

Dietician

Dieticians enable people to make informed and practical choices about food and lifestyle, in both health and disease. Dieticians provide advice on the best dietary choices for the person, to ensure that they absorb all the nutrients required by the body.
http://www.nhscareers.nhs.uk/details/Default.aspx?Id=189

Doctors

Consultants lead teams of doctors and specialize in a particular area, such as psychiatry of older age adults, paediatric orthopaedic surgery, dermatology or oncology (cancer). The team usually consists of senior registrars, registrars and junior doctors, often known as house officers. Newly qualified doctors have to undertake the foundation programme, a 2-year general training programme that forms the bridge between medical school and specialist training; they can be called F1s or F2s or junior doctors! There may also be medical students. Doctors may see patients and clients on a daily or weekly basis, depending on the nature of the placement. GPs are the only doctors you are likely to meet in a learning disability placement, unless the person is unwell and needs hospital treatment.

Summary

It can take a time to settle in to a placement. There are lots of new people to meet and new things to learn. Do not be too hard on yourself, if you feel bewildered after the first day, or that it is taking you some time to settle. Always show willingness to do the things you know you can; be honest about what you do not know yet and ask for guidance. Above all take an interest. Elsewhere in this book a student has said you 'have to fake it a bit sometimes' and this is good advice. In the unlikely event you feel this way, remember, you will not be welcomed or accepted if you arrive at the front door of a placement giving the impression that you do not really want to be there and looking bored. Why should your mentor take an interest in you? Why should he search for interesting learning opportunities for you? It works both ways. Be professional. Tell yourself it is only 4 weeks (or whatever) and be open to the experience.

More positively, embrace the learning in the placement you are enjoying and see it as the first step into practice as progress towards your goal of becoming a registered nurse.

■ Top tips

- Plan your first day carefully; be punctual, show an interest (without being pushy).
- Do not leave a placement during your shift without telling someone where you are going.
- First impressions count. Get off to a good start.
- Eat something *before* you go to your placement.
- If there is an emergency or other urgent activity you may not get a break.
- Feeling faint because you are not looking after yourself properly is not helpful for others or demonstrating professional behaviour.
- Learn about and value the roles performed by members of the multi-disciplinary team.
- Model yourself on the best practice you see. Set high standards and aim to achieve them.
- If you do not know something, admit it and promise to find out.
- Never give a patient your personal details, mobile, home numbers or address.
- However well you get on and like them, patient and clients are not our 'friends' (see Chapter 16).
- Relax and enjoy the placement; it may feel new and strange and a bit bewildering at first. This feeling passes.

■ Online resource centre

 For a link to useful clinical guidelines go to **www.oxfordtextbooks.co.uk/orc/hart/**

■ Further reading

Holland K and Hogg C (2001) *Cultural awareness in nursing and health care: an introductory text.* Arnold, London.

NICE (2004): **http://guidance.nice.org.uk/CG20**

More about the four fields of nursing

Sue Hart and Debbie Roberts

The aims of this chapter are:

➤ To raise awareness about each field of nursing practice

➤ To help you understand some of the language used and how nursing care may be organized

➤ To provide advice and guidance to support you when in placement

This is a long chapter and structured slightly differently from the preceding chapters. Please read this *entire* chapter. Why? Patients and clients do not fall neatly into categories to 'fit' the fields of practice. Adults with learning disabilities sometimes go into hospital; mental health nurses need to know about physical assessment, so they can recognize ill health in their clients. Just because you will follow a specific field of practice in the future, does not mean that you can divorce yourself completely from the others. *Nurses have a duty of care to all patients they nurse.* (See Fact box.)

! Fact box

The NMC (2004: 18) state that: 'The CFP should provide the foundation for entry to any branch programme. Students should have experience of each designated area of practice (branch) during the CFP'.

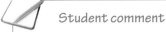

Student comment

❝ I think it is great if nurses in all areas understand about the roles of nurses working in different areas, to enable them to work together and complement each other. I think there is much stereotyping about mental health nursing, and I would say that having been on » placement I realize they do such an important job and that these stereotypes are not true!! I would encourage students starting the CFP to take the opportunity to learn about a different area of nursing while they can, as later on in the programme, in years 2 and 3, there is so much emphasis on what you *need* to know, naturally. It is nice to have a placement in an area that is interesting, but also knowing that this is not what you will be specializing in. 99

66 I think that a variety of placements in the CFP is crucial to gain an all-round picture of both mental and physical health needs. This will provide a good grounding for future practice, whatever branch, as you will encounter people with complex physical and psychological needs in all areas of nursing. 99

Important note

Some universities do not offer clinical placements for all fields of practice in year one, *only* those from your future branch choice. Irrespective of this, you may have to produce evidence that you *understand* the other areas; the following sections will help with this. Be aware that service provision varies within and across the four countries. The following can provide only a general overview.

11.1 Adult nursing

Adult nurses often work in NHS hospitals on the wards, in departments (such as accident and emergency), in outpatient clinics or a pre-admission unit (which screens patients before they are admitted for surgery). They also work in community-based settings, e.g. district (or community) nurses visiting patients in the own homes. Adult nurses work in small community ('cottage') hospitals or in walk-in centres or minor injuries units. Some are practice nurses based in a community health clinic or GP practice. Outside the NHS, many work in privately owned registered nursing care homes, or in independent special hospitals (such as the Royal Hospital for Neuro-disability in Putney) or private hospitals such as BUPA (**www.bupa.co.uk**). Nurses who specialize in palliative care are employed by hospices (see **www.pah.org.uk**). As Chapter 7 explained, your adult placement(s) could potentially be in any of these settings.

Finding your way around

Most general hospitals are organized according to body systems. For example:

- Respiratory ward (breathing).
- Gastroenterology ward (difficulties with digesting or absorbing food or elimination).
- Urology ward (concerns the urinary system).

They have outpatient clinics, as well as some specialist units (e.g. a pain clinic, day surgery unit). Most acute hospitals also have an accident and emergency department. *Intermediate* care services work between hospital and community. For example, if an older person falls at home, they may be visited and assessed by the intermediate care team to determine if a hospital admission was necessary, or whether the patient could be managed at home. Intermediate care services also help to organize discharge for patients either home or to other places, such as a nursing or residential home. Intermediate care is an expanding area for adult nursing. *Community* services care for a range of adult health needs, in a surgery (e.g. practice nurse) or in the patient's home (e.g. district nurse).

Being in placement in a hospital ward

Nightingale wards were set up in a military manner, and are long and narrow with beds on each side (see Figure 11.1a). Many of these are now being updated with partitions placed along the length of the ward to provide patients with more privacy.

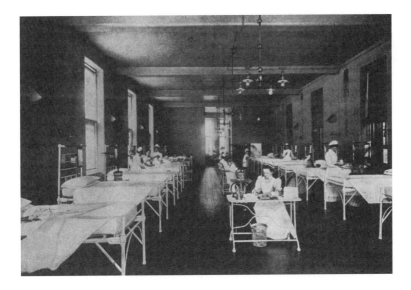

Figure 11.1a Old fashioned Nightingale ward © National Medical Library

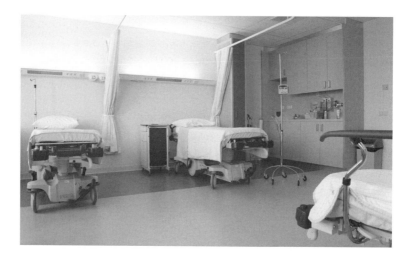

Figure 11.1b Modern ward © place to be/istockphoto

In newer hospitals, most wards are arranged in bays of two to six beds and have additional side (single) rooms (see Figure 11.1b). Certain wards consist only of single rooms, particularly if the patients need to be nursed in isolation, e.g. those with an infection. Newer wards will have piped oxygen and suction to each bed space, and many now have bedside television, radio and telephone, and even internet access facilities for the patient.

On the ward you will find:

- *The nurses' station* is a hub of activity containing the ward telephone, computer for access to patient results and/or patients' records and nursing notes, and emergency equipment, often referred to as 'the crash trolley'.

- Waste body products are disposed of in the *dirty utility* or *sluice room*. Here the contents of a bed pan will be flushed away and metal bedpans put through a bed pan washer. Cardboard bedpans go into a macerator (disposal unit). Dirty linen is also dealt with here. Used and soiled (e.g. if the patient has been incontinent) linen is placed in different coloured bags or 'skips'. You must find out what the procedure is on your placement.

- Some specimens are also tested in the dirty utility room (e.g. urine). You will find a *reagent cupboard* with all the equipment needed. There will also be measuring jugs, equipment for obtaining stool samples and other non-sterile items.

- Items known as *clinical waste,* such as used dressings and catheters, are disposed of in the dirty utility room, in special colour-coded bins, which are then incinerated.

- The *treatment room* is where sterile items are kept, such as new syringes and needles, gauze swabs, cotton wool and dressing packs. It is strictly for *clean equipment only.* Patient dressings may be done here (if not on their bed).

- The *drugs or medicine trolley* is often kept in the treatment room, locked to a wall. At various times of the day nurses dispense medication by wheeling the trolley to the patients' bedside. On the trolley (or in the treatment room) there will be a cupboard locked inside another cupboard to store *'controlled drugs'*. These (potentially addictive) drugs are used in pain relief and there are special guidelines governing how they are stored and administered. See: **http://www.dh.gov.uk/en/Healthcare/ Medicinespharmacyandindustry/Prescriptions/ControlledDrugs/index.htm**

- *Stores*: sterile equipment is kept separate from non-sterile equipment. You need to know where to find what you need, so check with your mentor and then have a good look around. Always ask before you open up sterile packets, usually the contents are listed on the pack.

- *Day room:* most wards have a provision for patients to 'escape' the clinical area to another room away from their bed.

Learning in an adult placement

What you will be doing when attending the placement depends on the type of area you are in. You may well be building on the skills you practised in the skills lab (e.g. observations) and have the opportunity to learn new procedures (e.g. dressings). In other areas the focus may be predominantly on the basic nursing care of patients: washing, assisting with food and fluid intake. It is all good learning for your future nursing career. Never think 'my friend on X placement is getting more experience than me'. It all evens out over the course of the programme. There is no such thing as a *bad placement*; it is all learning. Under supervision, participate as much as you can.

Learning away from the ward

In agreement with your mentor, be sure to experience as much as you can that is relevant to your placement, such as accompanying a nurse and patient to theatre, attending a pre-admission clinic or a discharge planning meeting.

Handover: nursing report

In an adult setting this event (introduced in Chapter 10) can take many forms. It may be given by one or more of the nurses on the previous shift, or by tape-recoded message. It may happen in a quiet room, at the nurses' station or at the patients' bedside. The information may be given in a particular order, which will vary from placement to placement. At first you may feel as though the information comes at you very quickly and that it sounds like a foreign language.

+

Nursing practice example 1 The language of adult nursing

On a surgical ward in an acute care NHS Hospital Trust you might hear something like this:

'. . . in bay one there's Mrs Jones, she's second-day following right THR, so she's for drips and drains out today and then for mobilization with physio. Taking sips and P'Uing fine so push fluids and we'll aim for catheter out mane'.

(Explanation at the end of this section.)

So that they understand what is being said, nurses tend not to use this type of language when talking with patients, but for your development, being able to *speak like a nurse* is important. Initially, not understanding can reinforce feelings of being a newcomer but do not panic. Gradually, as you become more accustomed to listening to the report, it will start to make more sense. Make notes and check out afterwards with your mentor.

? Stop and think

At handover, just listen carefully to what is said, rather than trying to write it all down. Later talk to your mentor about the meaning.

Mentor comment *Confidentiality in practice*

❝ You must ensure that your notebook *remains with you at all times* and is never lost, as it will contain detailed information. Destroy any loose papers at the end of each shift. You must maintain confidentiality at all times. ❞

See Chapter 15 for more about confidentiality, the Code of Professional Conduct and the NMC guidelines for documentation and record-keeping.

Student comment

❝ It's the abbreviations that are so hard to learn. I wish on every placement, as soon as you get started, that someone would give students a printout of all the different words that are relevant to that setting and the meaning of them. ❞

Also see the online resource for some more helpful vocabulary.

+ ....

Exercise 11.1

Start your own list of abbreviations used. Note the language used by staff. Is it respectful of the patients?

....

Who you may meet in an adult placement

Chapter 10 introduced many of the professionals who make up the multi-disciplinary team. You may meet some of them and also the following:

- *Staff Nurse*: a registered nurse. This person prioritizes, plans, delivers and evaluates the nursing care to a group of patients, and teaches students.

- *Sister or Charge Nurse:* an experienced nurse who leads the ward team. These people set the tone for the ward and are hugely influential in terms of being a role model; many are pro-active in teaching students.

- *A specialist nurse:* has done further education to practice at a higher level, e.g. in diabetes, cancer or cardiac care.

- *Healthcare Assistant (Auxiliary, Healthcare Support Worker):* These people work alongside registered nurses. They must undergo basic training in order to do their job. They are invaluable in caring for patients and families. You can learn a lot from healthcare assistants, especially in your first year and particularly with regard to basic nursing care skills. Always be respectful of the work they do and the role they perform. Registered nurses value the support of these staff members.

- *Ward Clerk:* helps the efficient running of the ward and knows what should be happening at all times. Answering the telephone, responding to queries, ordering supplies are all key activities.

! Fact box

You will need to familiarize yourself with the equipment on the crash trolley; to know what the equipment is for and how it will be used in an emergency situation.

The organization of nursing care

Some of the more popular methods of organizing care within adult nursing have particular names, like team nursing, task allocation and primary nursing.

- *Team Nursing* is where a group of nurses, healthcare assistants and students plan and deliver care to one group of patients with another team looking after others. Often the same group of nurses will care for the same group of patients each time they are on duty; this is referred to as providing continuity of care.

- *Task Allocation* is where each nurse undertakes a particular set of tasks for all the patients on the ward (e.g. blood pressures). Critics call this conveyor-belt nursing and believe it stifles 'holistic care' (care of the whole person).

- *Primary Nursing* makes the nursing care of a patient from admission through to discharge the responsibility of one nurse. The primary nurse co-ordinates care round the clock, planning the care to be given in her absence through associate nurses.

+ ....

Exercise 11.2 Primary nursing

Wright (1994) suggests that student nurses can act as *associate nurses*, so read up on this system if it is used on one of your clinical placements.

....

Writing about the care that you provide

You must record the nursing care given in the patients' nursing notes, or care plan. This may be electronic or hand written. Depending on the area you are in, a template with headings might be used for this based on the 'nursing process' or a care pathway (see more about these at **http://guidance.nice.org.uk/CG**). Student nurses must have their entries countersigned by a registered nurse.

! Fact box The nursing process/individualized nursing—key stages

- Assessment (finding out the needs of patient)
- Planning (planning how best to address the needs of the patient)
- Implementation (doing it)
- Evaluation (thinking about how well it went from both the patient's and professional perspective)

For more see Roper *et al.* (1996).

Community placement

A lot of adult nursing now takes place in community settings. Depending on the role of your mentor and your experience to date you may be either observing most of the time or be able to participate in certain aspects of care. This will be irrespective of whether you are placed in a community health clinic or with a nurse visiting patients at home. It is important to remember that nurses are guests in the home of their patients; you must respect this at all times and, as on the ward, display exemplary professional behaviour.

Student comment

66 I am doing adult now, but I loved working with the mental health community nurse, so much I considered changing branches. It was brilliant to observe how well my mentor could communicate with people, and I learnt a lot from her about talking to people who are very anxious and helping to calm them down, and cheering up and motivating people who were depressed, both very useful for adult branch! I also learnt a lot about dementia, I saw how nurses on the wards often called up the mental health team in the hospital to help with patients on the ward, when they could have dealt with the problems themselves with a bit of communication. So that was very useful. I also wasn't phased by a lady who went a bit nuts (sorry!) because of a UTI and started waving a walking stick at the nurses, because I had experience, and had learnt a lot through that. 99

■ Top tips

- Find out where the emergency buzzer is at each patient's bedside and know what it sounds like.
- Expect frantic activity if the buzzer sounds and respond if asked to help.
- Always follow instructions given by your mentor; ask if you do not understand, and never guess.
- Never carry out a procedure that you have been told you must not do.
- Always find out where the emergency exits and fire extinguishers are on every placement.
- Observe the uniform policy (to the letter). Looking 'right' will help you to 'feel' right.
- Do not wear your uniform outside the hospital (unless needed for a community placement).
- When on a community placement you are a guest in the home of patients. Value and respect this.

■ Online resource centre

 Want to learn more key terms and abbreviations used? Go to **www.oxfordtextbooks.co.uk/ orc/hart/**, where you'll find this and links to National Guidelines on Adult Nursing.

■ References

NMC (2004) *Standards of proficiency for pre-registration nursing education.* Standard 6, p.18. NMC, London.

Roper N, Logan W and Tierney A (1996) *The elements of nursing: a model for nursing based on a model of living.* Churchill Livingstone, UK.

Wright S (1994) *My patient, my nurse. The practice of primary nursing,* 2nd edn. Scutari Press. London.

■ Further reading

Holland K (2008) *Applying the Roper Logan and Tierney Model in practice,* 2nd edn. Churchill Livingstone.

■ Websites

BUPA (private health care organization): **www.bupa.co.uk**

Princess Alice Hospice: **www.pah.org.uk**

■ Answers

Answers to nursing practice example 1: The language of adult nursing

THR: total hip replacement.

Drips and drains: intravenous fluid drip and wound drain to be removed.

Mobilization with physio: physiotherapist coming to get Mrs Jones out of bed, ideally on her feet and taking some steps.

Taking sips: drinking small amounts.

P'uing: passing urine.

Push fluids: encourage drinking even more.

Catheter out mane: we plan to remove the tube through which Mrs Jones is passing urine tomorrow morning.

11.2 **Children's (or paediatric) nursing**

This field of practice involves everything from nursing a sick newborn to a teenager (usually up to 18) who has been in an accident. The challenges are varied (Glasper and Richardson 2006). Children's nursing is much more than caring for *miniature adults.* Children are particularly vulnerable because they are still developing. Also, most adults are able to articulate what they feel, e.g. the severity and nature of pain. Any child may struggle to communicate in detail and so nurses must interpret their behaviour and reactions; a very young (pre-verbal) child can never say what hurts. Also, a sick child can suddenly become very ill, so children's nurses need to recognize deterioration and respond instantly.

Children's nursing practice occurs in hospitals, daycare centres, child health clinics and in the child's home. Children's nurses work in NHS hospital settings, such as in paediatric or children's wards or children's accident and emergency departments. Others specialize in the care of the newborn and work in special care baby units (SCBU) or neonatal intensive care units (NICU). Community-based nurses' work with children with chronic and long-term conditions, such as cystic fibrosis, as well as those who are terminally ill and are being cared for at home by their families. You may attend child health clinics held in the community, e.g. where infants receive their childhood immunizations, or you may work alongside a school nurse visiting primary and secondary school children. Outside the NHS, children's nurses are employed in hospices (see **www.chasecare.org.uk**). The Children's Trust in Surrey (**www.thechildrenstrust.org**) provides care to children with multiple disabilities.

Depending where you are placed, *acute hospital* services for children may be organized according to medical and surgical wards and may be further subdivided according to age groups. Alternatively, where there is only one children's unit in a hospital, then there will children with a range of needs. So you could be nursing children with cardiac (heart), oncology (cancer), renal (kidney) or orthopaedic (bone) conditions in adjacent beds.

Some of the language of children's nursing

+··

Nursing practice example 2 The language of children's nursing

'Leslie Carbutt, aged 10 months, brought in to A&E by parents. H/O unwell past 2–3 days, diet, fluids, wet nappies. S/B GP yesterday, no active treatment. O/E flushed & febrile, T: 39 degrees C, Resps 28, Pulse, 120, SAO2 94. Audible cough, but otherwise quiet baby; for MSSU for CS, Bloods for FBC, U&E ?UTI.'

How much of this did you understand? At first such language sounds strange but with a little effort you will soon understand. Answers at the end of this section.

··

Other useful definitions:

- *Perinatal:* the time immediately before or after birth.

- *Neonates:* newborn infants (usually refers to the first 4 weeks of life).

- *Premature babies:* those born before 3 or more weeks before full-term gestation.

Mentor comment

66 *Don't expect to achieve anything in the first 2 weeks. Just get used to being in the world of children's nursing, watch and listen, absorb the atmosphere. Notice how we keep the atmosphere calm. Tune into this.* 99

! Fact box Parents and families

The parents of children in hospital normally have round-the-clock access to their child, and hospitals now provide facilities for parents to stay with their children overnight whilst they are in hospital. The facilities might be as basic as a recliner chair at the side of the child's bed through to a suite of rooms with kitchen and shower.

Facilities

Many of the facilities found in adult nursing environments (above) will also feature in children's wards. But particular to a children's wards are:

- *Play rooms:* most children, if they are able, will be out of bed and be spending time in the ward playroom. Even when children are unwell, it is natural for them to want to play. Children who are in hospital for a long period of time may even have lessons during treatment.

- *Milk kitchen:* many infants and small children will require breast milk or artificial milk formula for nutrition. It is vitally important that all the equipment in this area is clean and in some cases is kept sterile (feeding bottles, for example, will need to be sterilized), so milk kitchens are usually kept solely for this purpose and NO other activity. Breast milk can be stored frozen and so you might see a milk bank of frozen breast milk for infants. Formula milk can only be stored in a fridge for up to 12 hours. You would be expected to wash your hands thoroughly before entering, and wear a protective plastic apron over your uniform whilst you make up formula in the kitchen.

- *Beds and cots:* in all cases there will be a range of both cots (for infants) and beds.

- *Decorations:* children's wards are made to look much less clinical with colourful pictures, mobiles and other decorations on the walls, floors and ceilings.

- *Parents' rooms:* a designated space on a ward for families to take a few moments respite from the bedside of their child

The safety of children is paramount. Access into and from a children's unit is monitored at all times. The level of *security* differs from an adult placement, where it is usual, during the day, to operate an 'open-door policy'. As a junior student on a child placement you *may not* be given a key or swipe card of your own but have to ring a bell to enter the area.

Who you may meet

Many staff found in adult wards (healthcare assistants, radiographers, pharmacists, etc.) will also be present in children's wards. The following are a selection of specialists in working with children, who are members of the multi-disciplinary team:

- A *paediatrician* is a doctor who has done additional training to specialize in the treatment of infants and children. A consultant paediatrician will be an authority in a specific area of children's medicine or surgery, such as cardiac, gastro-intestinal or neuro-disability. They may also specialize in an age group, e.g. neonatal care.

- *Specialist children's nurses* have done additional learning to understand more about certain needs, such as growth (endocrine) epilepsy, oncology and diabetes.

> **! Fact box** Uniforms
>
> The trend some years ago was for children's nurses to wear *mufti* (non-uniform) often polo shirts and trousers. It was believed at the time that children would feel more comfortable with this casual appearance. However, virtually all areas have now reverted to uniform. It is felt that the presence of the uniform highlights the competence and professionalism of the staff and gives confidence to children and their families that they are in safe hands. It is also very helpful to identify who's who, which was one criticism of the non-uniform era.

- If it is considered that a sick child (and possibly also their family) may benefit from 'talking therapy' they may be referred to a *child psychotherapist* or a *child counsellor*.

- A *play therapist* works with young children, and occasionally adolescents, who have a range of psychological difficulties and complex life experiences. They may intervene where a child is having treatment for a life-threatening illness or a chronic long-term condition. Psychological difficulties may include depression, anxiety, aggression and attention deficit and hyperactivity disorder (ADHD). Difficult life-experiences include abuse, grief, family breakdown, domestic violence and trauma. A play therapist can help a child or young person to have insight into their difficulties, therefore easing internal conflict and building coping strategies. *Play therapists* work closely with a child's parents/carers, as well as other professionals.

- *Family care coordinator's* help, for example, by supporting a sick child when their family has to leave the bedside for a few hours.

- *Speech and language therapists* assist children who have difficulty producing and using speech, difficulty understanding or using language, difficulty with feeding, chewing or swallowing, a stammer or other voice problems.

> **! Fact box**
>
> A *dietician* will advise the child and their family about nutritional needs. If they are permitted to, it is important that children who are unwell eat and drink. Many parents' want to see on hospital menus healthy foodstuffs for their child. Conversely many children who are unwell just want comfort 'finger food', e.g. chips, fish fingers and sandwiches. This is sometimes an area of tension!

- *Parents' forums* are support groups for those who have children with long-term (chronic) or terminal illnesses. Here parents who are having similar experiences can get together to help each other through difficult circumstances. Some groups may be led by a professional; *self-help groups* are where families get together without this support.

Learning in a child placement

If you are open to learning, there is much to gain from a child placement. If you are on a children's unit you will be in practice under the supervision of your mentor caring for a small number of children, many of whom will have their family present. Note the comment from a matron on a children's unit about the activities you will be expected to undertake.

Mentor comment *(Matron)*

❝ What I have noticed is that first-year students seem to come to us from the university focused on their need to learn, which is great, but not always understanding that nursing involves things like, playing with children, talking with children and their »

> families, cleaning equipment (we must clean beds and lockers when children are discharged). Taking linen out *is nursing*. Keeping cupboards tidy *is nursing*. Students do need to see the whole picture. Nursing is not just *'procedures'*. "

You will come across children with various needs and with numerous conditions (Warner 2006). You are likely to meet some who have physical (e.g. cerebral palsy) or learning disabilities (such as Autism or Down's syndrome). You will learn all aspects of caring for children, as well as some special areas such as pain management and the use of pain-assessment scales. Sometimes you may nurse a child who is an inpatient for the duration of your placement; at other times they may have very short admissions with a quick turn around.

The organization of nursing care

Most areas will use pre-written and set care plans following the NICE (National Institute for Health and Clinical Excellence) guidelines.

Exercise 11.3

See the NICE website (**www.nice.org.uk**) and find more guidelines for caring for children with diabetes and other common conditions.

Vulnerable children

Sometimes adults do not care for children in the way they should or hurt them in some way. Being aware of this and understanding about safeguarding children is very important. Please see **www.everychildmatters.gov.uk**.

■ Top tips

- You need to be intuitive in order to sense how a child is feeling.
- Reassurance and encouragement of a poorly child is necessary.
- Read the non-verbal communication and respond to it with empathy.
- Always interact in a kind and caring manner.
- Keep calm—children sense when adults are frightened.
- Praise the child even for small achievements, make eye contact and smile.
- Immediately report any concerns about a child to your mentor.

- The ability to play and interact comfortably with a child is vital.
- Be open-minded, non-judgemental and enthusiastic about your learning.
- Registered children's nurses need the confidence to handle the distress of children and their parents in sometimes very difficult and sad circumstances.
- If you are going to be a children's nurse you will need to be confident to do the complex drug calculations required for children's medicines, without being reliant on a calculator.

■ Online resource centre

 For advice on what to do when working with vulnerable children follow the links at **www.oxfordtextbooks.co.uk/orc/hart/**

■ References

Glasper A and Richardson J (eds) (2006) *A textbook of children's and young people's nursing.* Churchill Livingstone, London.

Warner HK (2006) *Meeting the needs of children with disabilities.* Routledge, Abingdon, Oxon.

■ Further reading

Bee H (2006) *The developing child*, 11th edn. Addison Wesley, London.

Department of Health (2004) *National Service Framework for Children, Young People and Maternity Services.* HMSO, London.

Smith L, Bradstow M and Coleman V (eds) (2002) *Family centred care: concept, theory and practice.* Palgrave, Basingstoke.

Trigg E and Mohammed TA (eds) (2006) *Practices in children's nursing: guidelines for hospital and community,* 2nd edn. Churchill Livingstone, London.

■ Websites

Children's Charity Chase (hospice care for children): **http://www.chasecare.org.uk/**

Every Child Matters is a programme of change to improve outcomes for all children and young people: **http://www.dcsf.gov.uk/everychildmatters/**

Trust providing care for children with disabilities, at Tadworth in Surrey: **http://www.thechildrenstrust. org.uk/page.asp?section=00010001000400050001&itemTitle=At+Tadworth+Court**

■ Answers

Answers to nursing practice example 2: The language of children's nursing

A& E: accident and emergency.

H/O: history of . . . .

S/B: seen by . . . .

GP: general practitioner, i.e. own family doctor.

O/E: on examination.

Flushed: hot, red cheeks.

Febrile: feverish.

T: temperature.

C: centigrade.

Resps: inhalations of breath per minute.

SAO2 or SATS: oxygen saturation: the amount of oxygen contained within the blood, usually expressed as a percentage, i.e. out of a hundred.

MSSU: mid-stream specimen of urine.

CS: culture and sensitivity—the test done on blood for bacterial infection.

FBC: full blood count.

U&E: urea and electrolytes.

?: possible/likely

UTI: urinary tract infection.

And a few more you may hear:

PUO: pyrexia of unknown origin.

DIB: difficulty in breathing.

NAI: non-accidental injury.

HI: head injury.

11.3 **Learning disability nursing**

Learning disability nursing evolved from mental sub-normality and mental handicap nursing and has seen massive changes in service provision, the attitudes to service users and the roles of nurses. See the 'Valuing People' reports 2001, 2007 and 2009, which are available on the Department of Health website.

Today learning disability nurses mainly work in the community and support people at home who live alone, or with their families. Some areas have specialist treatment units for people with multiple disabilities or challenging behaviour. Some learning disability nurses have 'liaison' roles in acute NHS Trusts (supporting people with learning disability when they are admitted to hospital). Many nurses work in residential and respite services, usually now run by the social care sector or by the voluntary, independent or private sector.

Learning disability nurses aim to maximize the well-being of the person by improving their health and by enabling access to mainstream services.

Terminology

A learning disability is not an *illness*. When they need to, people access the health services as any other person does. Learning disability varies in its severity from mild and moderate, to severe and profound, with the most frequently occurring being Down's syndrome and autism (Watson 2007). Some people have an additional disability, e.g. sensory or physical. People's ability varies enormously. Many lead independent lives and have families and jobs. Those with medium support needs can function with the correct level of support for their needs. Those with very high support needs will require 24-hour care. If people are living at home, their families will often need support from statutory services, respite facilities and so on.

> **! Fact box** The health needs of people with learning disability
>
> This is a high-profile issue as many people have struggled to get the healthcare they need. See Hart (2007) and *Death by Indifference* (Mencap 2007) for more information.

Who you may meet

Community learning disability nurses work with children and adults and their families at home, or with paid carers in community settings. They are members of the MDT and are skilled to advise about and assess health concerns (through Health Action Planning). They may also advise about other areas such as behaviour and learning.

Psychologists in learning disability help with behavioural difficulties, such as, in the person best interests, to break problematic repetitive actions. This may be self-harming (e.g. gouging or picking at skin) or interfering with a person's ability to spend time in the community, e.g. touching people, which is not socially acceptable behaviour.

As the majority of learning disability services are now non-NHS providers, you will meet a *variety of different service providers* for your placements.

Many areas have *employment services*. It is the role of 'job trainers' to match people with learning disability to future employers and then teach the person the skills necessary to perform the job. Paid employment can help the person's self-esteem and enable increased independence.

Essential learning disability nursing skills

Sensitive interaction and good communication are key skills. Professionals need to be assertive to ensure people with a learning disability do not suffer discrimination. The work can be demanding, as progress can be slow. However, when someone has successfully learned a new skill you have taught them, the reward is tremendous.

Learning in a learning disability placement

A *residential service* is home for a small number of people with learning disability, which may be run by the local authority or an independent or voluntary agency. Today, they are run in a manner that is as 'ordinary' (i.e. non-institutional) as possible.

If the residents are fairly independent they may go out during the day to work or to a local college. In such settings most will be ambulant, mainly self-caring and be able to speak or make themselves understood using alternative communication systems such as Makaton.

In the house, others may need support to tidy their room, with bathing or training to boil a kettle. You will get involved in such 'ordinary' activities. Alternatively there may be the weekly shopping to do, someone to be accompanied to the dentist, others to a swimming pool, or for a walk. Some evenings may be spent at home, other times there may be a trip to the cinema or to a friend's party.

Nurse teacher comment

❝ It has been known that, when a student's placement has fallen during the time when the household were due to go together on holiday, the student has been asked to go along. Obviously this would be your decision. ❞

The learning opportunities are numerous. You will learn about the side of nursing that is not principally about 'hands-on' caring. Teaching new skills and supporting people to do things for themselves, are important parts of the nurse's role. You will learn about the lives of people with learning disability as you talk with them. Are they able to access services in the same way as you or I? If not, what are the obstacles? Ideally you will see how the staff members empower the people in their care to do things for themselves and how the risks of a person doing something new (e.g. crossing a road alone) are measured.

Mentor comment

❝ If you thrive on the hustle and bustle of an acute hospital environment, at times you may feel frustrated that you are not 'doing much'. Yet if you are open to the learning you can acquire knowledge, skills and values unavailable in a lot of other care settings and learn about yourself at the same time. ❞

In a residential service for people who have higher support needs your activities will be different. It is important that you understand what a person can do in order that they do all they can for themselves, and that their level of independence is maintained. The staff's role is to help the residents to do things they cannot easily do for themselves. The learning opportunities may include communication skills (especially non-verbal), management of epilepsy and incontinence, wheelchair handling, helping people to eat and drink, use of alternative therapies (massage, aromatherapy) and many more.

Some *day services* are still 'building-based', where people attend and do various activities (art, music, cooking). The newer day service provisions support people to use mainstream community facilities.

Community learning disability services: here learning opportunities may include working with a community nurse supporting a person with health action planning or teaching skills (such as travel training).

In a *'special school'* learning disability placement all the pupils will have learning disability and will be taught by 'special needs teachers' (and classroom assistants). An *integrated school* is a mainstream school that has an additional unit for special needs children. A school setting is an excellent placement to develop your communication skills (verbal and non-verbal) and to learn about teaching.

✛ ....

Exercise 11.4

If you have not already, visit the excellent resource: **www.easyhealth.org.uk.**
Watch the video-clips there to get a feel for the lives of people with learning disability.
....

The organization of care

Person-centred planning (PCP) approaches now feature across services. There are several types of these, three of which are summarized below.

> ! **Fact box**
>
> A 'person-centred' approach to care, places the service user (patient or client) at the heart of all nursing interventions, and sees the person as an individual with their own specific needs. Many contemporary services now adopt this philosophy of caring. Some critics of healthcare provision in the past have suggested that, prior to this, it was the needs of organizations or professionals that were centre stage. (See Ford and McCormack (2000) for more about person-centred care.)

Essential lifestyle planning (ELP)

ELP helps the understanding of what is important to the person with learning disability and can be used for people who have high support needs. By asking the person themselves (if they are able to communicate) or by asking others who know the person, the facilitator elicits basic information such as, What is the first thing you do in the morning? What happens if that does not happen? What do you do next? From such questions it is possible to build up a picture of what is essential to the person and what the person enjoys or prefers.

Individual service design (ISD)

ISD aims to bring about an increased understanding and awareness of the person and what 'makes them tick'. It asks questions such as: Who is the person? What do they need? What would have to happen to meet those needs?

Personal futures planning

This seeks to get to know the person and what their life is now, then to support them to decide how they would like their life to be in the future and help them to take action towards achieving this.

See Sanderson (2007) for more information.

Nursing practice example 3

A person centred PFP-type activity was undertaken with Doris (now aged 66) who, for many years, had lived in a long-stay institution, before she moved from there to a private residential service. Doris had a dream to have her own flat. Her advocate realized this and contacted a care manager. Within a year Doris had moved to a 24-hour staffed house, which is home to six people with learning disability all who live in their own flats.

How do you think the advocate managed to secure a place for Doris? Answer at the end of this section.

Exercise 11.5

If you are placed in a learning disability setting where person-centred planning is not taking place, ask why.

The language of learning disability nursing

- *Advocacy* refers to the role that professionals have in speaking on behalf of people with learning disability to ensure they get what they need.

- *Self advocacy* is where a person has learned the skills, developed the confidence, to speak for themselves.

- *Empowerment* literally means to give power. In learning disability services this means to encourage choice and decision-making and all other steps that move the person from a situation of dependence to one where they are more independent.

- *Normalization* refers to the idea that people with learning disability should live 'ordinary' lives with the usual variety (work, leisure, holiday) as other people.

- *Rights, independence, control and inclusion* are the key principles of the Valuing People directives (DH 2007, 2009) and are the goals that services should be aspiring to on behalf of service users.

- *Direct payments* means that money to purchase care is given directly to the service user and their family/supporters. The alternative is to pay for a person to go into an established service.

Exercise 11.6

People First is a national self-advocacy group. Visit their website: **www.peoplefirstltd.org.uk**. Note they prefer the term learning *difficulty* to disability. Reflect on why you think the NMC still use learning disability.

■ Top tips

- Communicate at the right level for the person.
- Learn about non-verbal communication (body language) and alternative forms of communication (Makaton).
- See the person and not the disability.
- Be kind and respectful, and listen.
- You do not have to be performing nursing 'procedures' in order to be learning.
- Join in activities.
- Talking with someone as they are doing their washing or while you are helping them to self-care can provide learning opportunities.
- Think about how you might work with a person with learning disability if you met them on another placement, e.g. mental health or acute hospital ward.

■ Online resource centre

Working with people who have learning difficulties for the first time can sometimes be daunting. For example, if your client has difficulty communicating it can be hard to ensure they are making the choices they want. For more advise and tips visit: **www.oxfordtextbooks.co.uk/orc/hart/**

■ References

Department of Health (2001) *Valuing people: a new strategy for learning disability for the 21st century* (Cm 5086). Department of Health, March 2001, White paper.

Department of Health (2007) *Valuing people now: from progress to transformation*: **http://www.dh.gov.uk/prod_consum_dh/groups/dh_digitalassets/@dh/@en/documents/digitalasset/dh_081041.pdf**

Department of Health (2009) Valuing people now: a new three year strategy for people with learning disabilities: making it happen for everyone: **http://www.dh.gov.uk/prod_consum_dh/groups/dh_digitalassets/documents/digitalasset/dh_094031.pdf.**

Ford P and McCormack B (2000) Keeping the person in the centre of nursing. *Nursing Standard* 46 (14): 40–44.

Hart S (2007) Health and health promotion. In: Gates B (ed.) *Learning disability: toward inclusion*, 5th edn. Elsevier, Edinburgh, chapter 15, pp. 281–300.

Mencap (2007) *Death by Indifference: following up the Treat me right! Report.* Mencap, London.

Sanderson H, Kennedy J, Ritchie P and Goodwin G (1997) *People, plans and possibilities: exploring person-centred planning.* Scottish Human Services Publications, Edinburgh.

Watson D (2007) Causes and manifestation of learning disabilities. In: Gates B (ed.) *Learning disability: toward inclusion*, 5th edn. Elsevier, Edinburgh, chapter 15, pp. 21–42.

■ Further reading

Gates B (ed.) (2007) *Learning disability: toward inclusion*, 5th edn. Elsevier, UK.

Hart S (2001) Spotlight on consent. *Learning Disability Practice* 4 (4): 14–17.

NHS Quality Improvement Scotland (2006) *Promoting access to healthcare for people with a learning disability, a guide for front line staff*: **http://www.nhshealthquality.org/nhsqis/1816.140.144.html**

■ Websites

Department of Health funded website to assist communication re health matters for people with learning disability: **www.easyhealth.org.uk**

Mencap, an organization supporting the well-being of people with learning disability: **http://www.mencap.org.uk/**

■ Answers

Answer to nursing practice example 3

The advocate, Janet, talked through with Doris what it would mean to have her own flat. They discussed how Doris would have responsibilities for her own safety, her front door key and her cleaning, cooking and laundry. As she would be living alone, Doris would have to go out to meet friends, or risk being lonely. Janet wanted to support Doris' wish, but was concerned she lacked the ability to live totally independently. Janet asked Karl (who owned the residential service Doris was currently living in) to host a person-centred planning meeting to discuss the potential move. Doris, Janet, Karl, Doris' old friend Belinda and Irena the care manager attended. Doris explained her dream, and with Janet's support, outlined her concerns. Karl agreed that Doris was no longer happy in his home and had asked to move. Belinda said Doris had often said to her that she wished to live alone. Irena explained to everyone about supported living arrangements, where a person could live in their own flat but still have 24-hour help at hand. Everyone agreed that this was a good option for Doris, and Irena promised to find out where there were vacancies.

11.4 **Mental health**

Student comment

66 I had a mental health placement in a dementia assessment unit and was dreading it before I went as I didn't know what to expect. I felt the value and purpose of this experience was to realize that people with dementia must be treated with the same dignity and respect as everyone else and they are usually frightened about what is happening to them and need reassurance. This will of course be extremely useful as an adult branch nurse, as we will be caring for people with these types of conditions throughout our careers. By the way, I absolutely loved this placement and really felt that I had helped to make a difference! 99

Whatever your future field of practice, you will come across people who have mental health difficulties. Recognizing some of the usual signs and symptoms, and understanding how people can be helped, will be useful for your future practice. Good nurses consider the 'whole' person. Roper *et al.* (1996) stress the *psychological* factors in all the 12 Activities of Living Model. As the student comment above shows, time spent in a mental health placement, or thinking about the needs of people with mental health difficulties, is valuable. There is a lot to learn.

> ! **Fact box**
>
> 'Service users', 'clients', 'residents', 'people' are all terms in common use in mental health settings. The word 'patient' is used sparingly. Nowadays, many services challenge the old-fashioned 'us' (i.e. professionals and paid carers) and 'them' (patients). Today mental health nurses practice *alongside* service users, teaching new skills and promoting mental health and acknowledging the part the person has in their own illness and recovery.

At any time approximately one adult in six has a mental illness (Dobson 1999). These range from common conditions, such as anxiety or depression, to schizophrenia, which affects less than one person in a hundred. Mental illness is not well understood and often still carries a stigma. Today most people are treated in primary care settings (Goldberg and Huxley 1992) and make a good recovery, with only a small number being referred to specialist mental health services. It is helpful to think about mental health services on a continuum from primary care to highly specialized services.

- *Mental disorder* is defined by the Mental Health Act (DoH 2007: 7) as 'any disorder or disability of the mind.'
- *Mental health or mental well-being* broadly refers to a person's ability to deal effectively with the challenges of everyday life.
- *The presence of a mental illness* is confirmed (diagnosed) by a psychiatrist. For more about specific mental disorders see the DSM-1V (APA 2000) ICD 10, or one of the websites recommended below.

> ! **Fact box** Mental Health Act Sections
>
> Most people seek help for themselves and are 'informal' patients who consent to being treated. A small number who are very unwell, and who may lack insight (awareness) about the severity of their difficulties, may be detained under a Section of the 1983 Mental Health Act. See **www.mind.org.uk/Information/Legal/OGMHA.htm** for more details. *Community Treatment Orders* allow for the person to be cared for in the community when their formal detention under a section ends.

Primary care	Specialized care
At home, in the community or GP surgery, by primary mental health care teams. This is how the majority of people with mental health needs are treated. People can access a range of health and social care services and voluntary sector (e.g. Mind) support.	Small number with enduring and severe mental illnesses need *specialist* input, in rehabilitation or acute admission units, and intensive support in the community.

Table 11.1 Illustration of primary care and specialized care in mental health.

Learning on a mental health placement

What you will be doing in practice depends on where you are placed. Your mentor will explain. Under the guidance of your mentor, take the time to enhance your communication skills, understand the world of mental health and learn about mental illness by being with the people who know best; the service users themselves. Observe and listen.

Who you may meet

Many professionals referred to in Chapter 10 as members of the MDT specialize in *mental health*. Others you may meet are listed below.

Mental health nurses

Nurses are often employed by mental health trusts. Many in specialist settings provide nursing care to people with serious mental health needs. Others work as *community psychiatric nurses*. Some specialize in patients with particular needs, such as eating disorders (e.g. anorexia or bulimia). Some mental health nurses work in the private sector.

What do mental health nurses do?

- Work in primary care mental health giving advice to other professionals and enabling referral on to specialist services.
- Nursing people with time-limited disorders (such as stress) by using treatments such as cognitive behaviour therapy (CBT) and counselling (more below).
- Nursing patients with more complex and long-term (enduring) needs who live in their own home or who are resident in mental health units.

> **! Fact box**
>
> Where possible, treatment occurs in a patient's home, at weekends and in the evenings, as well as during office hours. This can help to avoid hospital admission and helps support carers.

Clinical specialist mental health nurses

These nurses have particular expertise in one area, e.g. in dementia or drugs and alcohol. *Dual diagnosis* is the term used to describe people with a combination of drug and alcohol misuse *and* mental illness. Note also, that the term it is also used to describe people who have a learning disability and mental illness.

Approved Mental Health Practitioners (AMHPs)

These are qualified social workers, nurses, occupational therapists or psychologists who have done additional training to work with people with mental disorders and to carry out specific actions under the Mental Health Act.

Care coordinator (or key worker)

A member of the MDT, possibly, but not always a nurse, who takes the lead in coordinating the care programme approach reviews (DH 1999a) of the service users. Professionals in these roles usually have the most contact with the service user.

Psychiatrists

Doctors who specialize in the diagnosis and treatment of mental illness.

Graduate primary care mental health workers

Or, more recently, IAPTS (Improving access to psychological therapy services) are employed by GPs to manage and treat common mental health problems in all ages, including children.

Gateway workers

Link with GPs and primary care teams to support those people needing immediate or urgent help.

Learning in mental health placements

Student comment

66 I had a community mental health placement. I was very fortunate to gain excellent and extremely useful knowledge regarding mental health illness, issues and the services that are available out in the community. I have been very fortunate to be able to pass on this information to others. At first I was less than keen to do a mental health placement and was very blinkered about it. Yet I found that while I wouldn't want to do mental health as a future career, it has given me the ability to look at a patient as more of a whole rather than just look at their illness. From doing this placement I have since also been able to identify some patients that may have some mental health issues and help get them referred for the help they need. 99

The following indicates the types of placements that *may* be available for first-year students in either primary (first access) or secondary (rehabilitation and recovery) care settings.

- Working-age adults (up to 65 years) community mental health team (CMHT).
- Primary community mental health placement (PCMHT) assertive outreach team.
- Rehabilitation placement in a voluntary sector mental health service, inpatient or crisis service.
- Services for older people are normally organized to care either for patients with 'organic' conditions (such as Alzheimer's disease or other types of dementia) or for those with 'functional' conditions (meaning all other conditions expect for dementia). CMHTE community team for elderly people, inpatient units and residential care, NHS and private facilities. See DH 2009 for more about the latest in dementia care.
- Specialist services, e.g. children and adolescent mental health services (CAMHS). See National CAMHS Support Service (NCSS) website for more information **http://www.csip.org.uk/~cypf/camhs/national-camhs-support-service-ncss. html** and see the DAT website for more information **http://drugs.homeoffice.gov. uk/dat/directory/**

Exercise 11.7

Access the web pages of your local NHS Mental Health Trust to find out more about the services they offer, and specifically the type of placement where you will be attending.

- Community mental health teams (CMHT) are specialist multi-disciplinary teams providing assessment, treatment and care to people in their own homes and the community. They are usually made up of nurses, psychiatrists, social workers, psychologists and occupational therapists. The service will offer access to therapies such as psychotherapy and art therapy, as well as drug therapies (e.g. anti-depressants).
- Assertive outreach teams (AOT) work with people who have serious mental disorder, and are subject to care or treatment under a section of the Mental Health Act.
- Crisis teams work in an intensive way in a person's home to help them through a current period of acute mental ill health. They may intervene for as long as 72 hours and aim to prevent the person being admitted to hospital.

Therapies used in mental health

Nurse teacher comment

❝ Get to know the person rather than the illness. Think what you can do in the future to reduce the stigma and work positively with people who have mental illness ❞

- *Drug therapy* helps many people with serious mental illness by controlling their symptoms, e.g. for those with hallucinations (experiencing things like hearing voices that are not actually present) or delusions (false beliefs). For others, a short-term course of medication, e.g. to ease anxiety, can help restore good health.

- *Cognitive behaviour therapy* uses cognitive (thinking) techniques, such as challenging negative automatic thoughts. This helps people to explore their thought processes and consider how to re-interpret their experiences.

- *Psychoanalytic therapies* identify conflict arising from early experience that is being re-enacted in adult life producing mental health difficulties. The therapist aims to resolve this through establishing a rapport with the person and providing new opportunities for emotional insight. This is often a long-term process.

- *Family therapy* focuses on the interactions within families and aims to develop personal and interpersonal ability to enhance relationships.

- *Counselling*, through talking, gives individuals an opportunity to explore, discover, and clarify ways of living more resourcefully, with a greater sense of well being.

Exercise 11.8

Many other types of therapy are practised in the NHS including cognitive-analytic, existential, humanistic, feminist, personal construct, art therapy, drama therapy, transactional analysis, group analysis and interpersonal therapy (IPT). Find out more about these and how they can help.

Nursing practice example 4

Gavin, an office worker since he was 17, is now 26 years old and lives at home with his widowed mother and six cats. He has always experienced low self-esteem, mild depression and found it difficult to make friends but, despite this, he has held down a good job and worked hard. His mother is very domineering and controls his life as if he were still a child. In the past 2 years Gavin has sought comfort in over-eating and his weight has increased to a body mass index (BMI) of 29, which is bordering obese. (Search BMI at **www.nhs.uk** for more information.) Last week Gavin overheard colleagues giggling and making unkind comments about how he looked. Despite trying to keep his feelings hidden, it was too much. Gavin broke down and sobbed uncontrollably. His manager sent him home and said he must see his GP.

What do you think can be done to help Gavin? Answers are at the end of this section.

The organization of care

From April 2009, the National Mental Health Development Unit (NMHDU) has been the lead agency to implement new mental health policy priorities. Prior to this it was the National Service Framework for Mental Health (DH 1999b) which led developments. See the Department of Health website for the latest details.

Exercise 11.9

What pathways of care are in use in your placement? The care programme approach *must* be used for certain clients. Why?

- *Care Programme Approach (CPA)* people, who require specialist mental health services, are nowadays cared for using a model known as the CPA. This approach requires a care coordinator, a written care plan and reviews by the multi-disciplinary health team (DH 1999b).

- *Empowerment and recovery models* focus on the strengths of those with a mental illness to manage their return to good health by helping them to minimize the disabilities associated with their condition.

Exercise 11.10

Consider the ways that 'everyday' experiences (stress, sadness, anger) may come to be defined as 'mental health problems'. What do you think is the value to society as a whole of promoting mental health?

■ Top tips

- Go with the pace of the environment; accept you may not be 'busy'.
- Value the experiences of all people on the placement.
- Silence is OK.
- Be respectful and kind.
- Take people seriously.
- Observe the skills your mentor uses when interacting with the service users.
- Accept that you will often not know what to do or say; just listen.
- Report any concerns to your mentor.

■ Online resource centre

 For links to more advice from the Department of Health visit: **www.oxfordtextbooks. co.uk/orc/hart/**

■ References

American Psychiatric Association (2000) *Diagnostic and statistical manual of mental disorders (DSM-1V)*. American Psychiatric Association, Washington DC, USA.

Department of Health (1983) *Mental Health Act*. HMSO, London.

Department of Health (1999a) *Effective care co-ordination in mental health services: modernising the care programme approach*. HMSO, London.

Department of Health (1999b) *The National Service Framework for Mental Health: modern standards and service models*. HMSO, London.

Department of Health (2007) *Mental Health Act*. TSO, London.

Department of Health (2009) *National Dementia Strategy for England*. TSO, London.

Dobson F (1999) *Introduction to Department of Health National Service Framework for Mental Health: modern standards and service model*. HMSO, London.

Goldberg D and Huxley P (1992) *Common mental disorders*. Routledge, London.

ICD-10 *The International Statistical Classification of Diseases and Related Health Problems*, 10th revision version (2007): **http://apps.who.int/classifications/apps/icd/icd10online/**

Roper N, Logan W and Tierney A (1996) *The elements of nursing: a model for nursing based on a model of living*. Churchill Livingstone, London.

■ Websites

AllPsych online, see for more about mental health disorders: allpsych.com/disorders/dsm.html

Online resource to learn more about psychiatric disorders: **http://www.psychiatryonline.com/**

Website of the mental health charity Mind: **http://www.mind.org.uk/**

Department of Health (2002) *Dual diagnosis good practice guide*: **http://www.dh.gov.uk/en/ Publicationsandstatistics/Publications/PublicationsPolicyAndGuidance/DH_4009058**

Department of Health National Specialised Services Definition Set on web: **www.doh.gov.uk/ specialisedservicesdefinitions/index.htm**

The Sainsbury Centre for Mental Health: **www.scmh.org.uk**

■ Answers

Answer to nursing practice example 4

Gavin was still very tearful when he saw his GP the next day. The GP recognized that Gavin's situation was difficult and that he needed help. He said that, although anti-depressant medication may be helpful in the short term, in the longer term it could not help Gavin make the changes he needed to in his life. The GP gave Gavin a medical certificate for 4 weeks away from work and referred him to a nurse therapist for a course of cognitive behaviour therapy (CBT).

Bill, the therapist, saw Gavin later that week. They agreed they would meet twice a week for 20 sessions. Bill explained that through discussions they would look at Gavin's difficulties in terms of thoughts and behaviours and that, where necessary, Gavin could learn new techniques or ways at looking at himself and his life. Bill said they would focus on the 'here and now' and not delve too deeply into the past. He said he would sometimes give Gavin 'homework' where he would do things, such as test his beliefs and then change his behaviour to see what happens.

Four weeks later Gavin is keen to return to work, although the therapy will continue. He is no longer tearful. With Bill's support Gavin could recognize his difficulties and is beginning to understand that he can make changes in his life. He has started a weight-loss programme and has joined a support group with others in his situation. He also attends the local gym where he has made a new friend. Next week he is seeing a housing association about a rent-to-buy scheme. He has enough money for a deposit on a one-bedroomed flat.

Understanding reflection and reflective practice

Sue Hart

The aims of this chapter are:

➤ To explain reflection in a way it can be understood

➤ To help readers see the value of refection

➤ To give guidance to support reflective writing

Once you are in the second year (if not before) you will be expected to engage in *reflective* activities. When you write reflectively it is more than just description; you involve your personal feelings and thoughts and show an awareness of your actions. For many students (not through any fault of their own) reflection and *reflective practice* are much misunderstood terms. This misunderstanding is a concern, as both are *essential tools* to support personal and professional development.

12.1 What is reflection and why is it so difficult?

How you will be introduced to reflection and how you will be required to use it, will vary according to where you are studying. Some teachers introduce reflection early in the programme, others consider that it is a difficult concept and believe understanding it is aided by your experiences in theory and practice (i.e. when you have *something to reflect about*). What follows assumes the reader to have no prior knowledge of reflection. It aims to de-mystify (explain in plain terms) reflection. Please start by working through Exercise 12.1.

Exercise 12.1

Imagine yourself in 5 years time .... You have successfully completed the pre-registration programme and gone on to a variety of nursing roles. You have done a lot of continuing professional development (CPD) activity in your chosen field. Today you are at home preparing for an interview next week for a senior post, with a good salary and a lot of responsibility. For your preparation you try to anticipate the *qualities the interviewers will be looking for in the candidate they appoint*. What do you think these qualities will be?

This is a difficult question for you to consider at this point in your programme, and hard to answer because the interviewers will be looking for a range of skills, knowledge and experience. However, fundamental for them will be that they appoint someone who has obviously *grown and developed* in their practise since they first registered. How will this person (hopefully you one day!) have developed?

Do you anticipate in 5 years time you will be practising (e.g. undertaking a routine nursing procedure with a patient) in exactly the same way that you did last week when you were out in your placement? Will you have practised the same skills year after year with little development? Or will you be able to talk through how your practise has developed? The activities of reflection and reflective practice are essential if you are going to achieve the latter.

12.2 **Reflection defined and unpicked**

There are five definitions of *reflection* in the Concise Oxford Dictionary (1995), none of which capture the meaning of reflection in nursing practice. Surprised? It may help you to know that some academics believe that the word 'reflection' is not particularly helpful and this may explain why some students find the concept difficult. Biggs, for example (2003: 7) contends the word reflection is not the best choice to describe this activity. However, he adds that this should not detract from the value of the activity itself. He says:

> When you stand in front of a mirror what you see is your reflection, what you *are*. By contrast, 'reflection' as we are using it here [e.g. in nursing] is rather like the mirror in *Snow White* (a classic children's story with a 'talking' mirror): it tells you what you might be. The mirror enables the transformation from the … *what-is* to the more effective *what-might-be*.

Some years ago Boyd and Fales (1983, in Palmer *et al.* 1994: 13) proposed a definition *of reflection* which is still helpful today. They say reflection is:

> The process of internally examining and exploring an issue… triggered by an experience, which creates and clarifies meaning in terms of self, and which results in a changed conceptual perspective.

To aid your understanding we have unpicked the statement:

> The process of internally examining and exploring an issue…

This refers to a series of steps taken (process) to look at and question oneself (internally examining) by thinking and weighing things up (exploring), with the aim of learning from the issue.

> Experience…

Reflection needs a focus. For example, it will be about an *experience,* an incident or interaction that you have had, such as a conversation with your mentor or a patient.

Creates and clarifies meaning…

Questioning yourself later about the experience, chewing it over in your own mind, prompts you to think afresh (creates) and to come to see the episode clearly for what it was (clarifies). For example, you may understand an incident from the other person's point of view more clearly than you did at the time.

Self…

This activity leads you (self) to recognize, and give you insight into, the part you played in what happened.

Changed conceptual perspective…

Taking time thinking about the experience from your own and other's points of view can lead you to understand what happened, and why it happened, quite differently from before (i.e. a *changed conceptual perspective*).

Student comment

66 I found reflective writing a struggle to get my head around at first. I actually failed the first piece of reflective writing that I submitted due to getting too wrapped up in the act of reflecting and going off course regarding the subject that needed to be written about. I found it quite helpful to focus on one example of a reflective model, i.e. Gibbs (1988) rather than confusing myself further by looking at lots of different types. I think the biggest breakthrough I had in relation to reflective models was not to be scared of them, that they are only a tool designed to aid reflective writing and that they can be used as loosely or rigidly as you require. From being totally overawed by reflective models at the start, I have now come to recognize that they can help tremendously when analysing and reflecting upon practice. They certainly help to provoke ideas on how my practice and clinical skills can be changed and improved. 99

12.3 **So what is reflective practice?**

The word reflection describes the process (as in the definition above). When nurses are actively 'doing' reflection, they are engaged in *reflective practice*. Schon (1991) believes there are two main ways this happens: reflection *in* action and reflection *on* action. The goal of both is the same: they seek to promote an individual's development and learning by enhancing self-understanding in relation to an experience that has occurred. The difference between them is the time when the reflective practice takes place.

Reflection *in* action occurs at the time when the 'experience' (incident, episode, etc.) happens, e.g. *while the nurse is practising*. This prompts the process of reflection, as described above. Reflection *in* action is a *high-order* (highly competent, expert) skill, as in such a situation a nurse is required to 'multi-task' (i.e. to perform several skills at *the same time*). For instance, she may be reflecting on something the patient just said, doing a dressing (using fine motor skills), conversing with person (communication skills), comforting them (demonstrating empathy), explaining the procedure (teaching) and reassuring the patient that they should soon be ready to go home (empowering, confidence building) *all at the same time.* Who said nursing was easy!

Reflection *on* action, by contrast, is retrospective (i.e. after the episode has taken place) and for student nurses new to reflection, this is the best way to approach it. In such a situation, after the event, reflective practice requires that you go over what happened.

12.4 How may reflection be used on your programme?

Teachers use reflection in student nurse learning in a variety of ways.

Reflective assignment

You may be asked to write a reflective assignment, e.g. Based on administering a medicine under supervision, with the evidence-base for practice and demonstrating how patient safety was maintained (1000 words).

Reflective diary/journal

You may be asked to keep a diary of you reflections. This may be for your own personal use or you may be asked to let your personal tutor read extracts from it, which you will then discuss.

Reflective conversations

These can help widen your perspective and enable you to look deeply into situations, e.g. the wider implication of your actions (see Chapter 14). It can help you notice your strengths and, as a result, build confidence. Your personal tutor may engage you in reflective conversations.

Nurse teacher comment

❝ I am always upfront with students about reflection and say that some of them may find it hard, but that they *all* have the ability to do it. Like with any skills, for some it comes naturally, others have to work at it. Once they start, I remind them not just to reflect on things that go wrong or are difficult. I say reflect on your successes as well. Work out why something went well, so you can build on it. I also explain that *learning to reflect* as we teach students bears little resemblance to how they will *do* it later in their career. As when learning a new language, they may expect to stumble from time to time, later they will be more fluent. At first you write things down, later it is more of a cognitive, thinking activity. I suggest they build reflection into every-day life, like I do. When things have gone well in class I have reflected on why and then used those techniques again. ❞

12.5 **Starting reflection**

Reflective assignment

As with any assignment, you need to plan. Start as always with identifying key words.

A *written reflection* on *administering a medicine* under supervision with the *evidence-base for practice*, and how *patient safety was maintained*.

Most important: this is a reflection (not an essay or care study, as discussed in Chapter 6). *Write it as a reflection*. Read your guidelines with regards to the use of the personal pronoun ('I'). If 'I' is permitted, use it. If you are using a *reflective model*, e.g. Gibbs (1988), and are required by your teachers to write under the subheadings, plan which part of the answer below will fit where (see Figure 12.1).

You will be writing about your practice as, under supervision, you administered a medicine. *Briefly* described what happened. Where were you in placement? Who was the patient? What was the medicine? Why did they need it? How did you feel about what you were doing?

What do you *know* about administering medicine correctly (the evidence-base for your practice)? How do you know it? How did you know that you were practising correctly? Did anything go wrong? What was good about your practise? What was less good? Show that you are weighing this up in your mind (i.e. being analytical). If you made a mistake say so, and show how you have learned from it, and why you will know to act differently in future; for example, by demonstrating that you know what the NMC say about the safe and effective management of medicines and that this is one of the five essential skill cluster domains (NMC 2007).

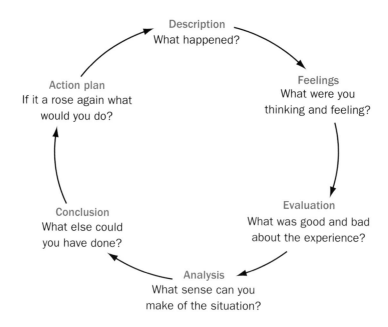

Figure 12.1 Diagram of Gibbs (1988) reflective cycle

What do you *know* about patient safety? Was it maintained and if not, why not? How did you know that you were practising correctly? Did anything go wrong? What was good about your practise? What less good? Again, if you made an error say so, and show how you have learned from it and why you will know to act differently in future and not make the same error again.

Conclude by summarizing what you have written and show you have learned from the exercise. Make sure you *reference* the correct administration of medicines and patient safety information.

··· A word about Models of reflection

These are intended to be helpful and to give you a framework on which to base your work. If you are asked to use a model, follow it carefully and relate your experience under the headings, as the student below has learned to do to her benefit. See some examples at the online resource.

Student *comment*

66 Reflection is a worthwhile task as there is a lot of information out there to discover and I have always found that when I do a piece of work like a reflection, I learn a lot. I am not sure that I have still grasped reflection fully—although I average marks »

in the 60s so I guess I'm not going too wrong! There is information 'out there' on how to write reflections, which can be useful, but probably the best bit of advice would be to break the work down into sections, write about these sections individually, then piece it together so that it makes sense and comes together in a fluent manner. 99

Reflective diary/reflective conversation

If you are *not* asked to use a model (whether you are writing the reflection or speaking to someone), it will help to consider (below) the work of Holm and Stephenson (in Palmer, Burns and Bulman 1994: 57). Ask yourself:

- 'What was my role in the situation? Did I feel comfortable or uncomfortable? Why?
- What actions did I take? How did I and others act?
- How could I have improved the situation for myself, the patient, my mentor?
- What can I change in future?
- Do I feel as I have learned anything new about myself?
- Did I expect anything different to happen? What and why?
- Has it changed my way of thinking in any way?
- What knowledge from theory and research can I apply to this situation?
- What broader issues for example, ethical, political, or social arise from this situation? What do I think about the broader issues?'

If you are writing a reflective journal, then use these questions to record your thoughts and feelings about the topic. If you are meeting your tutor, then you could use this list to prompt yourself and help you to get the most from the discussion. It would also show your teacher that you are developing your ability to reflect, which can only be a positive for you.

Remember, unless you are given a topic, you can select any area for reflection. It could be an incident where things went wrong. But remember, you can reflect on good practice as well as the less good. An excerpt from a real student reflective diary can be seen in Figure 12.2. This last piece of student advice is helpful as well.

Student comment

66 *I'm not sure that there was a time when the 'penny dropped'. I think it was, for me, more of a gradual process, and certainly I can look at my earlier work and see how much I have improved. I guess the old saying of practice makes perfect is true!* 99

17th Sept-

Was it better than I expected? I'm not sure. Just different issues I guess. After 3 hours of sitting alone reading a book of policies and procedures – all that meant nothing to me – I was told to go and meet clients. So out I went.

Everyone was really kind to me – the clients that is. They seemed delighted to have someone come and talk to them and make contact. Apparently staff don't sit and talk to them, as they are too busy. That's how my day progressed – just left to get on with it. The only thing is as I have no idea what I'm supposed to be doing I just sat and listened.

I heard a lot of frustration today. One lady got all dressed up ready to go out for her afternoon walk, only to find her escort has disappeared (I'm not allowed to accompany any clients). Another eagerly awaiting her O.T. to discuss bank issues and other stuff, but the O.T. didn't show up. Someone else was telling me how she normally came in voluntarily but because her CPN 'wasn't around' the last time, she had been sectioned.

Figure 12.2 An excerpt from a student's reflective diary: first day in a mental health placement

■ Top tips

- You can learn to reflect. If it does not come naturally—practice.
- Reflection is difficult to teach. It is not always your fault if you do not understand straight away. Stick with it and ask questions.
- If you want to be a good nurse grasping the basics of reflection is important.
- See reflection as a tool for aiding your development.
- Learn to enjoy reflection; it is your opportunity to say what you think.
- Keep all your reflections. Re-read them in a year or two or even later. They may make you smile as you will see how far you developed.

■ Online resource centre

 For examples of reflective models visit: **www.oxfordtextbooks.co.uk/orc/hart**

■ References

Biggs J (2003) *Teaching for quality learning at university.* Open University, Buckinghamshire.

Boyd EM and Fales AW (1983) Reflecting learning: key to learning from experience. *Journal of Humanistic Psychology* **23** (2): 99–117 cited in Palmer A, Burns S and Bulman C (eds) (1994) *Reflective practice in nursing: the growth of the professional practitioner.* Blackwell Science, London, p.13.

Concise Oxford Dictionary, 9th edn (1995) Oxford University Press, Oxford.

Gibbs G (1988) *Learning by doing: a guide to teaching & learning methods.* Further Education Unit, Oxford Polytechnic.

Holm D and Stephenson S (1994) Reflection—a student's perspective. In: Palmer A, Burns S and Bulman C (eds) (1994) *Reflective practice in nursing: the growth of the professional practitioner.* Blackwell Science, Oxford, chapter 4, pp.53–62.

Schön DA (1991) *The reflective practitioner,* 2nd edn, Temple Smith, London, cited in Reflection with a practice-led curriculum, chapter 1, p.13, in Palmer A, Burns S and Bulman C (1994) *Reflective practice in Nursing.* Blackwell Science, Oxford.

■ Further reading

Jones C and Freshwater D (2005) *Transforming nursing through reflective practice,* 2nd edn. Blackwell Science, Oxford.

NMC (2007) *Essential skills clusters.* NMC, London.

13

Assessment of clinical practice and portfolio development

Debbie Roberts

The aims of this chapter are:

➤ To introduce some of the ways your clinical practice will be assessed; the process and the paperwork

➤ To give guidance about writing learning agreements and building your portfolio

➤ To get you thinking about *evidence*

This chapter will explain the structure (i.e. some of what your portfolio will contain) and process (i.e. the usual steps) in the assessment of practice. It will outline the need to provide *evidence* of your activities through which you confirm that you have achieved all the required learning outcomes. Assessment of practice is an activity students undertake with their mentor; it is a collaborative process. It is not something done in isolation from you. When completed, this paperwork is placed in a folder that becomes your portfolio of practice evidence. Remember, the assessment of your practice accounts for 50% of the programme requirements, so it is essential to get it right if you are to be successful.

Important note

All university nursing departments across the four countries devise their own assessment of practice documentation according to what is required by the NMC and where they are (e.g. Wales practice requirements). The following terminology may not be an exact 'fit' where you are studying. However, you will quickly be able to glean what is what as you read the chapter, and look at the paperwork you have been given and follow your own uni guidelines.

Broadly, the key issues to think about in your assessment of clinical practice are:

• How are you going to achieve all you need to achieve?

• How are you going to provide evidence that you have achieved?

- How will your skills development be assessed in practice by your mentor?
- What will you put in your portfolio?

> **Mentor comment** *Explaining assessment of practice*
>
> 66 This is hard in a few lines but what I would say is that you should identify the learning outcomes you must achieve in the placement and your own learning goals/objectives, record them in a learning agreement/contract between you and your mentor, then engage in practice activities where you can meet the goals. Gather evidence that you have met the objectives/outcomes and place them in your portfolio. Add any other things you know you must, like reflections, orientation sheet. Then I will sign my bit, the student takes it to the university to submit (on time) for the teachers there to read, and sign their part. 99

13.1 How are you going to achieve all you need to achieve?

Learning agreements

Your learning agreement is the vehicle though which you meet the practice learning outcomes. You agree your learning goals with your mentor (in some cases your nurse teacher as well) and say what you wish to learn in the placement. Mentors expect you to input this as it shows your engagement in your learning. In reality both you and your mentor will make some suggestions, then agree and document this. If you are new to nursing you cannot be expected to know the full range of opportunities a placement in for example a minor injuries or rehabilitation mental health unit will have to offer. Talk to your mentor.

Examples of personal learning goals

- To learn about cognitive behaviour therapy (CBT) and observe a nurse using this technique with a client.
- To observe and then practise an aseptic technique.
- To accompany a person with learning disability to an outpatient appointment, to observe the medical staff communicating information about a health need.

- To observe a multi-disciplinary team discharge meeting for an older person.

- To participate in the process of a patient being taken to theatre and returned to the ward.

- To observe a nurse doing an assessment of mental capacity and then making a best interests decision. (DCA 2005)

You will be assessed on the outcomes of the learning agreement you have made with your mentor. As the above shows, the content of the learning agreement will vary from student to student.

Date agreement set	Learning agreement	Student responsibilities and goals	Teacher/mentor responsibilities	Evidence of achievement	Review date
1st January	To improve awareness of preparation of patients for surgery.	To attend 2 days observing in pre-operative nurse-led clinics. Listen to what patients say about coming into hospital for an operation. Speak to mentor about best practice in preparing patients for surgery.	To direct the student to relevant literature. Link teacher: to visit the student on placement and discuss progress. Mentor: to ensure student has the opportunity necessary to achieve the goal and to organize suitable days for the student to attend the clinic.	Following pre-op clinic visit, student will compile a checklist of key points that are relevant to the topic. Also to discuss at midway meeting. Pre-op nurse to sign summary of her 2-day visits.	Midway through placement.

Table 13.1 An example of a learning agreement between a first-year student nurse and a mentor and link teacher.

! **Fact box** How a learning agreement enables practice outcome achievement

Learning goal agreed: To observe a multi-disciplinary team discharge meeting for an older person who wishes to live independently again.
Would help you to achieve the following:
Practice learning outcome: Identify the roles of the members of the health and social care team, and participate in multi-disciplinary care delivery.
Evidence of achievement: Student notes written following the MDT meeting (preserving confidentiality); record of the visit to the social work department; comment from a case manager student shadowed for the day. Also, when asked by a mentor the student shows a good understanding of the role of the occupational therapist (OT) and discharge planning team.

Student comment

66 Plan your learning agreement having read through all the practice learning outcomes. Make sure what you want to learn will provide the evidence you need to meet the outcomes. Visiting a shelter for homeless people may help you to achieve outcomes in a community placement, but you may struggle to make it relevant on a surgical ward. Keep it in mind for another time. 99

13.2 How are you going to provide evidence that you have achieved?

Some more examples of evidence

- Your mentor observes you performing certain essential skills and confirms (in writing) that you are proficient to the level required of a first-year student.
- Your mentor writes a formative and summative report confirming you have achieved.
- You provide written evidence of your activities and how they met the outcomes.

You might include entries from your learning diary, specially selected to demonstrate your development, or perhaps some reflective writing, which links theory and practice together. Some placements will have organized study days or sessions for you to attend. The certificate of attendance for these can be used as evidence, accompanied by a few paragraphs saying what you learned from the session and how you will use the information or new knowledge and skills in your future practice.

• • • **A word about** Evidence

Remember from Chapter 6, evidence can take many forms. Here it refers to the work that you produce for your portfolio, which confirms to the marker that you have achieved what you needed to for the placement. It may be your mentor writing and signing a report about you, your learning outcomes signed off, etc.

13.3 How will your skills development be assessed in practice by your mentor?

The assessment of practice *process* describes what you and your mentor (and/or nurse teacher) have to do in order to complete your assessment of practice. To put it another way:

- *You*, under supervision, and through learning agreements, have to develop the required level of nursing skill or other activity (e.g. professional behaviour) in order to meet the outcomes for that placement and then, demonstrate your achievement through collating *evidence* in your *portfolio* for your mentor, future mentors and nurse teachers to read, and for you own record of your development.

- *Your mentor* must supervise you, and ensure you have sufficient experiences in practice in order for you to achieve your outcomes. They must support you to develop your learning agreement. They must provide on-going support and arrange at least two more formal meetings: a formative (midway) and summative (almost at the end) assessment of your practice. If you are struggling to achieve, there is also action they must take (more below).

Each mentor will have their own way of managing the assessment of student learning. Most will observe you performing a nursing skill and will assess you, discuss any issues with you, and provide you with feedback. Some placements may ask other qualified staff to also monitor your performance, with your mentor collating all the views and verifying your practice. Some mentors will tell you at the end of each shift the things that you have dealt with well or areas where you need to use alternative strategies. There are pros and cons to each of these but you should ask your mentor what kind of approach is used within the placement so you can prepare yourself.

At the end of the placement your mentor will *sign* to confirm you have achieved the practice learning outcomes and you will also have to sign. There will usually be space for comments from you both.

! Fact box Practice assessment

Remember, it is your responsibility to ask your mentor to undertake your practice assessment documentation in good time. Try to avoid leaving it until the last minute: plan ahead and get organized. If your mentor is unavailable you may need to see the nurse in charge of the ward.

Never be tempted to forge your mentor's signature. Such behaviour when discovered (it will be discovered as universities are alert to this possibility) ultimately will lead to you being removed from the programme.

··· **A word about** Action or development plans

This is a constructive and helpful activity to get you 'back on track'. You will meet your mentor and the liaison/link teacher, or even your personal tutor, to identify specific areas you need to address in order to achieve the summative assessment. This would occur when formative assessments have identified areas for further development. A further action plan would be necessary should you not achieve a pass at the summative point of the module.

Formative (midway) assessment in practice

These terms are both used to describe the meeting that takes place between the student and the mentor about half-way through the placement (see Figure 13.1). Your progress is reviewed and documented. By conducting this assessment half-way through the placement, you will have an opportunity to address any areas for concern. Remember that you also have to maintain the good practice that you have already demonstrated. Proficiency has to be demonstrated all the time, not forgotten about once you have achieved.

When a student is not doing well in practice, it can be for a variety of reasons. Examples are given below. (See Chapter 14 for more about professional behaviour).

Failing to achieve the learning outcomes

- This may be because you have been assessed as not yet competent, or may not have experienced a particular aspect of care in which you can demonstrate proficiency.
- Your mentor may have assessed that you are incapable of ever becoming competent. This means that there are concerns regarding your fitness to practice.

Failing in professional behaviour

- Persistently late.
- Not following instructions.
- Breaking confidentiality.

Mentor comment

❝ Lack of interest, knowledge and skills, are all reasons why students fail practice. Also, they fail when they do not demonstrate the necessary professional behaviour, but this is not usually until they have been told, prompted, reminded, encouraged. If they still cannot do it, then it is right they leave and do not join the profession. ❞

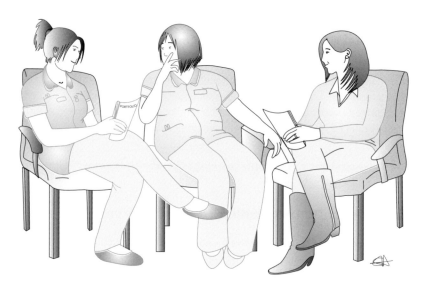

Figure 13.1 Three-way meeting: such a meeting is sometimes called a triangulation of assessment

What if you are not doing well in practice?

Student comment

❝ I was referred in practice early on, once. I was doing the obs and a patient had a very low BP. I knew I should tell someone but I got distracted and then forgot. The patient became quite unwell. I felt awful about it. I have *never* forgotten anything important again. I hope my *experience stops this happening to you.* ❞

You should meet regularly with your mentor to discuss how you are doing and, if the mentor feels that you need to work on certain specific areas of your practice, these can then be discussed. Remember that your mentor is there to help you to achieve but she does not have to pass you and indeed should *not* pass you if there are concerns about your practice. *When assessing students, registered nurse mentors are the gatekeepers to the profession.*

You might struggle with a particular placement for a whole range of reasons; some to do with the placement or the type of nursing that happens there and some to do with personal reasons or things that might be happening at home. If you don't think you are doing well in

··· **A word about** Fitness for practise concerns

At any time, if your mentor is concerned about your progress or development, a specific development plan may be put in place in order to help you to achieve the standards required. In order to write the development plan your mentor may ask your personal teacher to attend the meeting and/or a student representative (from a professional body or union, or you can ask a friend). Concerns raised are wide and varied, but you should be aware that if you do not achieve the elements within your development plan or the outcomes for the placement, you may be asked to re-learn a module of theory and subsequent practice, or you may be asked to withdraw from the course if the fitness for practise concerns are not addressed.

clinical practice, then you need to talk about it with your mentor or personal teacher. They can help you develop your knowledge, skills and behaviour or attitudes in clinical practice in order for you to achieve your learning outcomes. Meeting regularly with your mentor means that you will be fully aware of any concerns she might have about your practice and will be given the best opportunity to address these areas of concern.

Summative (final) assessment in practice, mentor final report on your practice

This is the final event to 'sign you off' at the end of the placement, hopefully having passed. Your progress is documented against the required outcomes and personal learning outcomes. Your mentor will complete all the paperwork, as above, and confirm in writing that you have achieved. You are advised to be vigilant that they have done it all. It is *your* assessment after all, and they are only human. Also, be careful to fill in all the details you need to for your part of the assessment; your comments are important.

Nurse teacher comment

" If your uni requires a personal teacher to verify aspects of your assessment in practice before you submit it, remember that you may need to make an appointment with them in advance, in good time, in order to meet the deadline for submission of your practice assessment documents at university. "

Nurse teacher comment

" Students often quickly tune in to the need to submit their essays and other written assignments on time but do not always realize that the same rules apply for their assessment of practice. There will be a date and time it has to come in. One minute late is too late. "

! **Fact box** Warning! Keep your paper work safe ready for the 'sign-off mentor' at the end of the programme

A sign-off mentor verifies that you have achieved *all the outcomes for the entire programme at the end of year three.* This *final* sign-off mentor role is determining that you are 'fit for practice' as a registered nurse. In order for the final sign-off mentor to verify your competence, you need to have evidence that you have achieved all the learning outcomes and proficiencies for the entire programme. You will be advised how this will be done.

13.4 **What will you put in your portfolio?**

Student comment

" You are soon forgotten! You may think it's OK to go back for a signature, but as soon as you have left, there is someone else to take your place and your mentor's time is taken up elsewhere, so always get things signed whilst on placement! "

Your portfolio is a record of your achievements and also a plan for your future learning and development. Your portfolio will demonstrate that you are able to assess your own development, identify what your learning needs are and plan how you will address these learning needs. The portfolio allows you to evaluate the learning that has taken place. In other words, it is a constantly evolving document. In summary, portfolios are designed to enable you to:

* Demonstrate your achievements during the module.
* Record your development through the programme.
* Prepare you for your future career (see below).

When you have completed the programme and are registered with the Nursing and Midwifery Council, you will need to maintain evidence of your continuing professional development through a portfolio. As we said in Chapter 1, the skills you develop in the programme prepare *you for your career*.

How you develop your portfolio and the various components that you will need to include will be determined by the requirements of your university and the module or unit you are undertaking. Wherever you are studying, the portfolio will need to be taken back to the university to be read by the nurse teachers and confirmation of your result notified to the examination office.

Nurse teacher comment

66 At my university the student portfolios are still on paper. Some universities are now moving to e-portfolios. We are in discussions about this at the moment. Students just need to do what is asked of them wherever they are. 99

In Chapter 9 we gave you examples of the assessment of practice paperwork you need to take into practice for your assessment. See the online resource for a copy of this to remind you in each placement of what you need to do. Chapter 9 also alerted you to how learning occurs. Once you are in practice it is important to understand what you need *to do* in order to provide the *evidence* that will satisfy your mentor and nurse teachers that you have successfully met all your objectives.

Whatever placement or clinical setting you are in, you will always have to provide *evidence* for your portfolio. The types of evidence will remain constant as shown below, irrespective of whether you are in an adult, child, learning disability or mental health setting.

Signed-off practice learning outcomes

In each case you must convince your mentor that you can consistently achieve and work at the standard required, so it is not just a one-off. You must show that once you have achieved the standard required, that you continue to apply that knowledge, skill and attitude throughout the programme.

••• **A word about** Practice outcomes covered by theory

Sometimes certain outcomes will have been covered by the content of lectures. If your assessment of practice has such outcomes, you will be told who will sign these off.

Observed structured clinical examination (OSCE)

On some clinical placements you may be required to undertake an OSCE (see Chapter 8). You may be tested on your communication skills or have to undertake the admission of a patient. See the online resource for OSCE tips.

Ongoing achievement of practice record (OAR)

As a student you are required by the NMC (2007b) to have an ongoing achievement of practice record, which goes with you to each placement. Your mentors from each placement will write comments about your progress relating to the NMC learning outcomes and your own personal goals, and will help you to identify future actions for your development. You are responsible for ensuring that you take your record with you to each placement and you are expected to share the record with your personal teacher at the end of each clinical placement.

Information to support your initial orientation to the placement

Mentor comment

66 You will be given a checklist of activities you must do on the first day, such as to find the fire exits, and will be made aware of what you must read as soon as possible, e.g. fire, manual handling, resuscitation, health and safety policies. Be sure to do all this and get it signed off by your mentor early on in the placement. 99

The do's and don'ts in practice

Most placements have policies for what students can and cannot do and you *must* follow such guidelines wherever you are. Helping you to know what you *should* and *should not* do is quite a tricky business, particularly as there is no one definitive list of things that students can or cannot do. So you need to think quite carefully about what you are being asked to do. For example, see Exercise 13.1.

Exercise 13.1

A staff nurse asks you to take a medicine pot containing several pills to Mrs Jones and to make sure she takes them. Meanwhile the nurse goes in to the next cubicle to give another patient her medicine. What should you do?

Now on the face of it, this might seem like a really simple task and a reasonable request. However, as a student you are *not allowed to administer medicines without close supervision*. This means that the staff nurse is responsible for ensuring that the correct patient receives and takes the correct medication; not you. In such a case politely (and quietly) and gently remind the nurse that you need to be supervised whilst administering medicines, and you know that this means she must *watch you do it*. The nurse will then sign the prescription card to say that the drug has been given with no adverse side-effects. *Never administer medicines to a patient without a registered nurse being present.*

Skills development record

This is a record of the skills in which you have been asked to demonstrate **competence** and will be based on the NMC essential skills clusters domains. Depending on your university, this may be a separate document or integral to your main assessment of practice. The essential skills clusters domains are:

- Care, compassion and communication.
- Organizational aspects of care.
- Infection prevention and control.
- Nutrition and fluid management.
- Medicines management.

See (NMC 2007) and the online resource.

Professional behaviour records

This records your performance with regard to the professional behaviour, which you must show you have achieved (e.g. correct uniform worn, suitable appearance, punctual). See Chapter 15 for more guidance about professional behaviour.

Mentor/co-mentor/associate mentor signature records

This is self-explanatory and will normally be cross-referenced with mentor specimen signature records held at the university.

Record of attendance/time-sheet

On-going records of hours worked and/or absences are necessary for you to provide evidence that you have worked the necessary hours required by the NMC in the first year. It may, depending on the circumstances, sometimes be possible to make up short periods of absence before your placement ends.

Where longer absences have occurred, these must be discussed with your personal tutor.

Record of night duty

Currently, nursing students are required to complete a minimum of 60 and a maximum of 230 hours of night duty during the entire programme. These hours must be recorded and confirmed by your mentor. Most of these hours are done after the first year, once you have moved into your field of practice study.

Visits and short-placement evidence

Generally, a visit is no longer than 1 day, a short placement is about a week, as part of a longer placement. Remember all placements should be for a minimum of 4 weeks. In both instances you need to have identified learning goals and have a learning agreement, which will then be completed as evidence for your portfolio.

Observation of your practice record (direct observation)

When presenting an observation as evidence in your portfolio, it must show your knowledge of the theory underpinning your actions, in other words demonstrate that you can link theory to practice. For example, your mentor could observe you helping the person to eat a meal. You then write up what you did, how you did it and why. Your mentor signs to confirm this happened.

Additional evidence

Include paperwork evidence to support any additional activities you must perform, such as keeping a reflective journal, submitting reading logs (see Chapter 6 and 12 for more about these).

Check-list for successful portfolio building

- Always read your own university portfolio completion guidelines with care and do *exactly as you are asked.*
- When in practice, keep your learning outcomes and the need to provide evidence of them for your portfolio at the front (not the back) of your mind.
- Work steadily on your portfolio every week. Do not wait until the last week to start work on it.
- Make sure you complete and submit *all* the aspects required in your portfolio on time. You cannot be successful if you omit required content.

- Where your portfolio has a space to write your name, sign your name, or give other information, such as placement name, dates attended. Make sure you mentor does the same.

- Do not let your mentor take your portfolio home with them (it is your portfolio, guard it carefully). If they leave it on the bus what are you going to do?

- Always be present when your mentor is 'signing you off'.

- Use only relevant evidence; be selective about what you put in.

- Show that in practice you also are thinking about theory and your professional development and provide evidence for this. For example, refer back to articles or books you have read when in placement. Note examples of professional behaviour you have witnessed.

- Your portfolio is marked on quality not quantity. Do not write more than you need to; keep your focus.

- Information pamphlets that you have picked up in practice are not evidence of anything! A friend may have given it to you and you may not even have read it.

- Never *ever* leave a placement for the last time without your portfolio paperwork complete.

13.5 **Your assessment in practice; possible outcomes**

Depending on your performance in clinical practice, there are various outcomes that could follow:

- *Pass or achieved*: the outcomes have been met and the student has demonstrated consistent performance against the proficiencies and outcomes.

- *Partially achieved*: means some (not all) outcomes have been achieved. With more practice, the student is likely to achieve the required standard. Following this outcome, a detailed action plan is usually drawn up to highlight exactly what is expected in terms of further development by the student in order to achieve the required standard. Your personal teacher may attend the meeting and help to formulate and agree the action plan.

Not achieving in practice (refer or fail)

If you are unable to achieve all your learning outcomes, you might not pass the assessment of practice. This is called different things in different universities, e.g. it might be known as 'being referred in clinical practice' or 'failing clinical practice'. Being referred means that you have not met all the learning outcomes, this does not mean necessarily that you have not met *any* of the outcomes, as you may have been referred in only some. So, if you are referred in clinical practice, it should not come as a shock, because your mentor will have discussed your progress with you at regular intervals, long before the final formal meeting takes place. If you are referred in clinical practice *don't panic*! Students are usually given more time (although this may be limited to a few weeks) and a second attempt in order to achieve the learning outcomes and so improve the areas in which they have been referred. Remember that you have to pass the requirements laid down by the NMC in order to progress in to your chosen branch. If you are referred at the second attempt, then the university might expect you to undertake the module of learning and associated practice again, which might mean that you join a group behind you. The mechanisms for referral in practice should be well publicized and available through your examination and assessments department or on your university website, so make sure you are familiar with the system, both what is expected of you and what you can expect from the university and practice staff in terms of help and support. Ultimately, however, you should be aware that if you cannot pass the learning outcomes for practice, you may be asked to withdraw from the course.

In *exceptional cases*, where there are concerns over fitness to practice, a student may be suspended from the clinical placement whilst a full investigation takes place. Fitness for practice issues are very serious, but are always dealt with in a professional manner. Issues can range from doubts about occupational health, through to gross misconduct. Issues relating to fitness for practice may or may not include the application of disciplinary action against you.

> **! Fact box** NMC 12-week rule
>
> In case of any difficulties, the NMC allow up to 12 weeks after the end of the common foundation year in which to achieve the year-one outcomes. But aiming to achieve within the year is always the goal.

13.6 **Assessing your practice portfolio**

Once you have handed in your portfolio at the university, it will be marked and moderated (see Chapter 5) by the nurse teachers and will go through the usual exam board processes. You should be made aware of the result in the same way as you would a theory assignment.

13.7 **Evaluation of your practice**

Both the placement and the university always want to know what you thought about your time in a placement. Did you learn? Were you well supported? If you have had an enjoyable and useful placement with a supportive mentor, then it is kind to say so and thank everyone. Your mentor will be pleased to hear such a comment, however many students they have had. Back at the university, when evaluating practice in discussion and on paper, be careful always to be honest and professional in your comments.

Student comment

66 When we got back from our first placement our tutor went round the class and asked for our opinions. Generally everybody had a bad time (they thought) but had all come out with excellent grades because we had sought out learning opportunities. This taught me a lot. 99

Summary

It is your assessment of practice. Others are there to help but you have to achieve. Alert your mentor, link or personal tutor to any difficulties you may be having, as soon as they happen. They are there to help and want you to succeed. Be open about any areas that you find difficult, so you can get the help you need. Do not avoid situations that you know you have to achieve.

■ Top tips

- Your assessment is a collaborative process; your mentor should not make judgements about you without discussion with you.
- Double-check if they have missed anything and ask them to address it.
- Ask your mentor to start the summative assessment of practice at least a week before you are due to leave to avoid mishaps (e.g. your mentor being off sick on your last day).
- The more you engage in your learning the more successful you will be.
- Refer to the portfolio check-list above every time you have to submit a portfolio.

■ Online resource centre

 To help you act on the advice in this chapter and develop your portfolio ensure you visit **www.oxfordtextbooks.co.uk/orc/hart/** where you will find examples of the assessment of practice paperwork, and links to the NMC outcomes for entry to the branch including the Essential Skills Clusters. Make sure all you have learnt is conveyed well by looking at the OSCE tips, also online.

■ References

Department for Constitutional Affairs (2007) Mental Capacity Act 2005 Code of Pratice. The Stationery Office, Norwich, UK.

NMC (2004) *Standards of proficiency for pre-registration nursing education*. Standards 02 04. NMC, London.

NMC (2007a) *Essential skills clusters*. NMC, London.

NMC (2007b) *On going achievement of practice record*. NMC, London.

■ Further reading

Kozier B, Erb G, Berman A, Snyder S, Lake R and Harvey S (2008) *Fundamentals of nursing. Concepts, process and practice*. Pearson Education, Harlow.

Nairn S, O'Brien Elisabeth, Traynor V, Williams G, Chapple M and Johnson S (2006) Student nurse's knowledge, skills and attitudes towards the use of portfolios in a school of nursing. *Journal of Clinical Nursing* **15** (1): 1509–1520(12).

While, A (2003) Learning ought to follow mistakes. *British Journal of Community Nursing* **8** (2): 96.

The profession of nursing

Sheila Muller

The aims of this chapter are:

➤ To help you understand what a profession is and what it means to be a professional

➤ To help you understand the work of the Nursing and Midwifery Council, the professional body for nursing

➤ To help you understand what is meant by professional behaviour in placements and at university and why this is important

➤ To give you strategies to support your developing professionalism

The book so far has made you aware that to be successful you must achieve in *all* the three areas: theory, clinical practice and professional development. Being skilled in two of these areas, but not the third, is *not an option*. The following two chapters provide you with a foundation on which to build your understanding of what it means to be a professional, and *how to behave professionally*. It builds on the content of previous chapters and is the last link in *the theory–practice-profession model* we introduced at the beginning of the book.

The previous chapters have mentioned professional behaviour several times. In Chapter 5 the issue of professional behaviour in lectures; Chapter 8 noted that contacting your placement *before* you start is considered good professional behaviour. As you read on, you will sometimes see overlaps and links back to content that has been touched on before. *To see this as repetition is to miss the point.* The point *is* that the theory, practice and professional skills overlap; they do not exist in isolation from one another. To be successful, you must understand this. When in *practice* registered nurses draw on their *professional* judgement and *knowledge* all the time. But, before we consider professional judgement and behaviour this chapter starts with a question.

14.1 **What is a profession?**

A profession is made up of people who are members of an occupational group who share a common body of knowledge and set of skills that have been gained through a formal course (e.g. a pre-registration programme), which has resulted in a qualification and registration as a member of that profession. As well as nurses, other professionals include lawyers, doctors and dentists.

As *high standards of behaviour and practice are at the core of every profession* there are expectations about how the people who call themselves 'professionals' should carry out their work, behave towards their clients and the public, as well as towards their colleagues.

Nursing is a profession that demands the public's trust and professional behaviour will be a central part of your theoretical and practice education. Your *integrity, trustworthiness* and *honesty* are very serious concerns for everyone working in the health services due to the implications for the safety of patients and clients.

+··

Exercise 14.1

Table 14.1 summarizes just some of the responsibilities of the members of a profession. Based on what you have read so far in this book, can you add to it? Try now. If you struggle, come back to this when you have read this chapter.

···

To be a *professional* means to uphold the standards of that profession at all times.

Obligations	• To serve patients, clients, families, customers.
	• To work on their behalf.
	• The competent and safe use of knowledge and skills.
Standards	• Must be upheld at all times.
	• Come from professional ethics, the law, policies and standards relating to our own professional integrity.
	• Respect for all people, regardless of ethnicity, religious beliefs, gender, sexual orientation, socio-economic background.
Responsibilities	• Lifelong learning.
	• Truthfulness and honesty.
Difficulties	• Conflicts between professional and personal life.
	• Coping with responsibilities.
	• Respect for personal and professional boundaries.

Table 14.1 Examples of professional responsibilities.

14.2 **More about the Nursing and Midwifery Council (NMC)**

The NMC is the regulatory (professional) body for nursing and midwifery. Doctors have the British Medical Association (BMA); the equivalent for nurses (and midwives) is the NMC. Every chapter in this book so far has mentioned the NMC. But what exactly do they do and why are they so important? The NMC exists to establish and improve standards of nursing and midwifery care in order to protect the public and it does this in a variety of ways. For example, it:

- Specifies standards concerning admission to training and the structure and nature of pre-registration nursing programmes.
- Sets standards for nursing and midwifery education, performance, ethics and conduct and provides advice and guidance on professional standards.
- Maintains a register of qualified nurses and midwives.
- Considers allegations of unfitness to practise due to misconduct, ill health or lack of competence.

Specify standards concerning admission to training and the structure and nature of pre-registration nursing programmes

The pre-registration programmes prepare students for entry to the nursing register. The NMC specifies standards concerning those it admits to training (e.g. qualifications, CRB, references). It also specifies standards for the *structure and nature* of pre-registration nursing programmes (see Chapter 2.2 if you do not understand).

In 1999 the NMC responded to concerns from practising nurses and nurse teachers that, on completion of the Project 2000 nurse education programme, students were not quite ready for practice as registered nurses. What followed was the Peach Report (1999) and the recommendation for the Fitness for Practice Curriculum. This built on the strengths of Project 2000, one of which of was to produce practitioners who were able to contribute to

---

! Fact box

Nurse education programmes must *also* fit the specific characteristics of higher education programmes (universities) in the content of the curriculum, and quality assurance (QAA 2001, 2002). Also its standards for education and training must satisfy European Community obligations.

service management and development, to embrace change and to be flexible with regard to working in many different healthcare settings, depending on their own career choices, and the needs of the NHS.

The NMC is concerned about the *good health and good character* of all those entered on the register; these are both absolutely essential to being a nurse. Good health means that you will be able to undertake the theoretical and practical aspects of your pre-registration programme. There is more about good character to follow.

· · · **A word about** Students with disabilities

People with disabilities are welcomed in the nursing profession and the Disability Discrimination Act (2005) means that everyone who has the capability to benefit from studying or working should be given the opportunity to do so. Your university and partner NHS Trust will have policies in place to ensure that it meets the requirements of the Disability Discrimination Act, to enable you to take a full part in university life. The broad policy aims are based on the Quality Assurance Agency (QAA) Code of Practice: Students with Disabilities and the Disability Discrimination Act (Parts 3 and 4) Code of Practice.

Set standards for nursing and midwifery education, performance ethics and conduct

The NMC code, which came into force in May 2008, spells out in detail the required standards of conduct, performance and ethics for nurses. Its principles are of key importance to you as a student in your own development and then as a registered nurse. It encapsulates what the people you care for and your colleagues should expect from you in your practise. *To help you in your developing professionalism the code is discussed in detail in Chapter 15.* As a student nurse, the standards set by the NMC are important to you.

At the time of writing, the NMC is consulting on a new *code of practice for student nurses* (more below) to replace the 'NMC guide for students of nursing and midwifery' (2005). The link to the new document is not available at the time of writing, but will be at the online resource for this chapter. You should always read such documents in conjunction with advice provided by your higher education institution (university).

Maintains a register of qualified nurses and midwives

The NMC has a statutory obligation to protect the public and to maintain public confidence in its registrants by setting standards to assure the quality of the people it registers as nurses. When you complete your pre-registration programme, your university will notify the NMC that you have 'met the required standards and you are eligible for entry on the register.' A declaration of good health and good character will be completed by your course

> **! Fact box** NMC Register
>
> This is the term used to describe the up-to-date record of all registered nurses held by the NMC. The register consists of two sub-parts for nurses. There also parts of the register for midwives and for specialist community public health nurses. The registration and entry codes are as follows:
>
> Adult: [RN1, RNA]; Mental Health: [RN3, RNMH]; Learning Disabilities: [RN5, RNLD]; Children: [RN8, RNC].

> **· · · A word about** PIN numbers
>
> PIN stands for Personal Identification Number and is your unique identifier in the profession. You pay every year to continue to be on the register and to keep your right to practice. If you are not on the register, you cannot practise as a registered nurse. The annual fee is currently £76.00.

director and sent to the NMC. Your sign-off mentor will also have confirmed that you have met the required standard in clinical practice. When that information has been received, and you have paid your registration fee, your name will be entered on the NMC register and you will then be able to practise as a registered nurse. The information about the registration of a nurse, midwife or other professional is in the public domain and can be checked by anyone.

Considers allegations of unfitness to practise due to misconduct, ill health or lack of competence

As you know, all nursing students are required to undergo a Criminal Records Bureau (CRB) or Disclosure Scotland check. This is because they will be coming into contact with vulnerable client groups, and the safety of patients is paramount in healthcare. The references provided for you by your school, college tutors or previous employers are also checked by the university before you are offered a place, to confirm your good character.

Your good character is very important as nurses must be known to be honest and trustworthy. Your character must be sufficiently good for you, as a student and then as a qualified nurse, to be capable of safe and effective practice without supervision.

On rare occasions, registered nurses *do not* meet the professional standards that are expected of them by the public and their professional colleagues. In these cases, the NMC investigates any complaints made about the professional conduct or competence of the person. This activity is just the same as it would be in any other profession that had cause to doubt a member's behaviour. You may have heard of doctors being 'struck off', i.e. losing their right to practise. The same can happen to nurses.

Overwhelmingly (99.8%) of registered nurses practise professionally and competently throughout their careers. Unfortunately just under 0.2% of registered nurses some time fall short of the high standards required. In such instances their conduct is investigated by the NMC Fitness to Practise Directorate. Sanctions imposed range from suspension to removal from the register.

Sometimes student nurses do something wrong, either by accident or (rarely) deliberately, and they are investigated through procedures at their universities. Examples of unprofessional behaviour include plagiarizing (see Chapter 5) academic work or another student's essay, or forging a mentor's signature.

Not only are these acts wrong in themselves, they suggest that the individual may feel that forging a signature on a patient's notes, or cheating by copying the work of others is somehow acceptable. Where next? Writing false information on records? Telling lies? Cheating in an examination? Stealing?

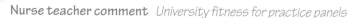

Nurse teacher comment   *University fitness for practice panels*

" One aspect of my role is to put the nursing department's case against a student whose behaviour questions their fitness to be on the course. We do spot-checks on portfolios and hold a bank of specimen mentor signatures, so we easily discover those who forge. I find it even worse when it is obvious that they have been found out but go on to lie and lie about it. I have never known anyone found guilty of forging a signature and not been told to leave the course. When they appear before the university fitness for practice panel I feel ashamed that such people would ever want to be nurses and pleased that we caught them early on, so they do not devalue my profession by becoming registered nurses. Please tell your readers from me: there is no place in nursing for dishonest people. "

Good students can worry about get things wrong *unintentionally*. Rather than fret, read the next section. It will guide you in all aspects of your professional behaviour as a student.

14.3 **Your developing professionalism**

Above and elsewhere in this book we mentioned the NMC Guide for Students of Nursing and Midwifery (NMC 2005). We have also indicated that at the time of writing the NMC are consulting on a new *code of practice for student nurses* (now available at the online resource). What follows has been informed by the original code, what we have seen from the consultation and many years of working with student nurses in practice and assessing professional behaviour. As you read, pause from time to time and make links back to what you have read about in previous chapters. This activity will help consolidate your understanding of what it means to be a *professional*.

The NMC student guide outlines the key professional aspects of caring for your patients and clients while you are a student. It gives guidance on the extent and the limitations of your professional accountability, and will help you throughout your pre-registration programme. As a new student you are most likely to be observing care being given, and as you go through your programme you will help in providing care. As a senior student you will have full participation in providing care to your patients and clients.

The principles that form the foundation of this guidance reflect the professional standards that will be expected of you when you become a registered practitioner, which are to be found in the code (NMC 2008).

Understand what is meant by accountability

+ ....

Exercise 14.2

Look up the words accountable and accountability in a dictionary. Think about what they mean and how the meaning applies to you as a student nurse in all aspects of your course.

....

If you have read the book so far you should by now understand that as a student, *you* are not professionally accountable in the way that you will be once you are registered. So far as the NMC is concerned, it is the registered practitioners with whom you are working who are professionally responsible for the consequences of your *actions and omissions* (see Fact box) and you cannot be called to account for your actions and omissions by the NMC. This is why you must always work under direct supervision. This does not mean, however, that you can never be called to account by your university or by the law for the consequences of your actions or omissions as a pre-registration student, and your professional skills and behaviour are as important as they will be when you are a registered practitioner.

Understand what is meant by the wishes of patients

As mentioned in Chapter 10, as a student, you must respect the wishes of patients and clients at all times. Although most people will be happy for you to help look after them, they do have the right to refuse to allow you, as a student, to participate in caring for

> **!** **Fact box** Actions and omissions
>
> In this context, *actions* are things that you did that you *should not have done*, e.g. taking money from the purse of someone with a learning disability without their permission; taking tablets from a medicine trolley for your own use; with holding food from a patient in a mental health setting who has been 'difficult'.
>
> An *omission* is where you *did not do something you should have done*, e.g. not recording the giving of medication at the time you gave it (i.e. contemporaneously).

them and you should explain this clearly to them when they are first given information about the care they will receive from you. You should leave if they ask you to do so as their rights, as patients or clients, supersede at all times your rights to knowledge and experience.

Understand why you should always identify yourself

You should introduce yourself accurately at all times when speaking to patients or clients either directly or by telephone. In doing so, you should always make it quite clear that you are a pre-registration student and not a registered practitioner. In fact, it is a criminal offence for anyone to represent him or herself falsely and deliberately as a registered nurse or midwife.

+

Exercise 14.3

Notice how your mentor and other staff introduce themselves to patients or clients or other professionals. Do they use first names, titles, and job or role title? Do they do it differently in different circumstances?

Understand what is meant by accepting responsibility for your actions

As we have said before, there will be times when you might not be directly accompanied by your mentor, supervisor or another registered colleague. As your skills, experience and confidence develop, you will become increasingly able to deal with these situations. However, as a student, you must understand *why* you do not participate in any procedure for which you have not been fully prepared or in which you are not adequately supervised. Seek guidance *now* if you are still confused.

Understand what is meant by patient confidentiality

Patients have the right to know that any private and personal information that is given in confidence will be used only for the purposes for which it was originally provided and not used for any other reason. For example, as we explained in Chapter 6, some of your assignments will be about the people you have cared for and you must not provide any information that could identify a particular patient or client. You should access patient records only when absolutely necessary for the care being provided. Use of these records must be closely supervised by a registered practitioner and you must follow the local policy on the handling and storage of records, which will be held in your placement area or as part of the local online resources. Any written entry you make in a patient's or client's records must be counter-signed by a registered practitioner. You can find more advice about confidentiality in the NMC code (2008). You should also refer to the NMC guidelines for records and record-keeping, which can be found on the NMC website and the online resource.

+ ....

Exercise 14.4

Think of some of the ways in which confidentiality would be broken in using technology to communicate with colleagues and friends.

....

You must not discuss your student colleagues, your placement colleagues and, above all, patients and clients when you are using sites such as Facebook, msn, or MySpace. Also, you must not use email or text messaging on your mobile phone to discuss anything that concerns patients or colleagues. It is easy to make a mistake, so be very conscious about how you communicate with friends and colleagues.

An example of how technology can be 'misused' occurred when a student nurse took some pictures on his mobile 'phone of a patient he had been caring for. The student then showed the completely ordinary pictures of the patient waving and smiling to qualified colleagues, who realized immediately that this was a breach of confidentiality. The 'phone was confiscated, and action was taken to ensure that this could not happen again. The patient was completely unaware of the risks involved in having his picture taken, and the student nurse felt very upset when he realized the implications of his action.

If you are ever worried that there has been a breach of confidentiality, then you must tell someone in authority so that the issue can be dealt with effectively. It is your duty as a professional to make sure that the privacy and confidentiality of everyone in your care is protected.

X **Avoid** Making promises you cannot keep

If a patient tells you something that puts you under a strain, such as they have not been swallowing their medication when given it, and then asks you not to tell anyone, you *must not* promise this. Your duty is for the well-being of the client. This over-rides any concern you may have that they may be cross with you for betraying their confidence. Asking you to keep such a confidence is unfair to you; do not let it compromise what you know is the correct behaviour. Tell your mentor.

Understand how to act if you see something you think is wrong

As a student, you will experience a range of different settings in your practice education placements. You will be well placed to question why something is or is not being done. In some cases, you may see a registered nurse or midwife doing something you feel is not correct. Although you are likely to feel that this places you in a difficult position, you should not ignore the situation. Initially, you may not feel confident about asking them personally or someone else about it. There may be a sensible explanation.

However, sometimes you may be observing something that could amount to misconduct. If you ask a registered practitioner about something they have done that you feel concerned about, and they respond in a helpful way, then you can feel encouraged that your questions show you are an observant and thoughtful student. If they respond defensively, then you should speak to the ward manager, your mentor or your tutor.

The NMC guide tells you what you must and must not do. Read on now to develop your understanding of what it means to be a *professional* and the duties and obligations that come with the role.

Understand what professional behaviour in placement means

In nursing, as in all professions, each individual is responsible for their professional behaviour. The principles of this apply to students as well as to qualified staff. The level of responsibility differs, depending on your individual level of competence, but at all levels you accept responsibility for your actions and omissions. As well as being responsible to yourself, and to your patients and clients, you are responsible to your profession to maintain high standards and integrity and not bring the nursing profession into disrepute.

As part of your professional behaviour, you are, as an adult learner, responsible for your own learning in order to improve standards of knowledge and practice.

Clinical placements are one of the most important parts of your education programme. It is only through placements that you get the opportunity to put all the theory you have been learning to use out in the 'real world' of practice, as well as to gain all the practical experience and skills that you need to learn and pass your pre-registration programme.

You should approach the clinical placement aspects of your programme with professionalism. The course is demanding and you will sometimes feel that the demands on you are overwhelming. Long shifts, with academic work to finish when you are off-duty, as well as trying to maintain your personal life, all mean that approaching all aspects of your course in a professional way will make it much easier for you to manage any issues as they arise, and will help you avoid running into problems.

Understand why punctuality and reliability matter

The work of the health services goes on for 24 hours every day. The nature of nursing means that patients and clients cannot wait for you to be ready at your own pace to care for them, and your qualified colleagues and your mentor will need to get on with caring for people, and cannot wait for a student to arrive. It is, therefore, 'professional' to arrive on time for each work shift or meeting with your mentor, and to be reliable when you have made arrangements with colleagues. Mentors have often said how stressful it is for them to be waiting for a student, either because they had arranged to demonstrate a particular clinical procedure, or because the student had arranged a specific assessment or discussion of an aspect of their portfolio. We all know what it is like to wait at home for a delivery that does not arrive at the pre-arranged time. We can't get on with other jobs, we can't go out and we feel that the company making the delivery has fallen short of behaving in a professional manner.

+..

Exercise 14.5

Think about ways to ensure you will always be punctual and reliable. If you have a genuine reason for being late, or are unable to get to your placement, then show your professionalism; ensure your colleagues are aware of your difficulties.

....

Understand why your appearance matters

As a learner, and along with your professional colleagues, you should always ensure that your appearance is suitable for attending placements, and university. This can be more complicated than it at first appears. As a new student, you might make the reasonable assumption that as a nurse, you will always wear your uniform. However, there are a number of placements where uniform is not worn, and you will be told that you can wear 'your own clothes'.

This *might* suggest to some of you that your favourite low-cut top or a very short skirt could be worn. This will not be acceptable. One way of thinking about what to wear when you are in placement but not in your nurse's uniform, is to develop an alternative 'uniform' of clothes that is suitable for every setting. You may decide to have extra pairs of black trousers and practical tops that you know will be suitable for placements that do not require you to wear uniform (e.g. those with health visitors), and that can be washed and dried far more easily than glittery T-shirts.

The over-riding message about your appearance with regard to clothes is that you should look professional and comfortable, so that you can get on with working in your placement without the distraction of impractical clothing.

Other aspects of your appearance are also really important, to mark you out as a professional. Your shoes should be comfortable, but even if you are ordinarily most comfortable in 4-cm stiletto heels, these are never suitable for placements. As previously mentioned, metal rings and other adornments need to be removed whenever you are on placements, although you can sometimes wear sleepers in your ears. It is usually acceptable to wear a wedding ring and a small neck chain under your uniform or clothes. If you are unsure of local policies, or your university policy on this, then make sure you have found out what these are in advance of arriving at your placement.

Your appearance is an important part of professional behaviour for reasons that relate to how you care for your patients. Such adornments are very likely to cause problems with infection control, as you move between patients, washing your hands, but unable to do this to the highest standards because of rings or bracelets. They may cause practical hazards to patients, such as scratching them as you care for them. They could also cause you injury, e.g. if you are helping a patient to move from their bed to a chair, your ring could get caught on equipment, and so injure your finger. So, from a practical as well as a professional point of view, least is best.

+ ···

Exercise 14.6

Imagine that you have booked a nice restaurant for a special occasion. You have sent out the invitations to your friends, and have written clearly that everyone must arrive on time, and be smartly dressed. On the day, two of your friends are late, as one got lost and the other one overslept. You and everyone else have been waiting, and so have the restaurant staff, as they can't start making your meal and serving it until all of the guests in your party have arrived. To make matters worse, another friend, who has arrived on time, has not stuck to the dress code for the restaurant, arriving in torn jeans and an old T-shirt, and looking as though they haven't washed for a week (perhaps they haven't). How do you feel? Upset and very let down because the three people who have not kept to the rules have ruined the occasion for you and everyone else, made you feel embarrassed and have disrupted the staff in the restaurant who are very busy trying to keep up with all of their customers.

Understand why good communication is important

We have alerted you before that it is good manners to contact the placement at least 2 weeks in advance of your starting date. If possible try and talk to your mentor, but always leave up-to-date contact details in case they need to contact you. Why is this important?

An example is that of a student named Ginny, who was informed that her placement would be in the community, based with the community nurses at a small local clinic. She was given the name of her mentor. She *did not* contact the placement in advance and leave her details, but arrived at eight o'clock on the first morning of her placement, expecting that there would not be any problems. When Ginny arrived, the building was closed and there was nobody around. She was puzzled and then concerned as to whether she had arrived at the right place. After waiting for a while, she telephoned the university placement office, and they gave her the contact details of other district nurses who were part of the same team. When she contacted them they said that her mentor was off sick, and as the mentor often worked alone, the building would be closed for the day. They said that they would have telephoned her to let her know of alternative arrangements, but that because she had not contacted them and left her telephone number they could do nothing.

Placement arrangements can sometimes change at the last minute. Hospital wards can close, mentors be off sick. There are numerous things that can happen on the first day to interfere with your placement. Making sure yourself that arrangements have not changed is the best action you can take.

+

Exercise 14.7

Put the number of the uni placement office in your 'phone *now* in case something untoward happens on your first morning and you need to speak to someone.

Understand how to manage your mobile 'phone when in practice and at university

Mobile phones are, for many of us, our main way of communicating with family, friends, colleagues and everyone else. We can all become very reliant on our mobiles working. Nevertheless, mobile phones must be switched off during academic teaching sessions because, at best, someone's specially chosen ring-tone is distracting, but it is bad manners for your colleagues and the tutor to have to put up with this kind of disruption.

Mobile phones must also be switched off whenever you are on placement, and may have to be switched off across a whole site. It is up to you to find out about, and adhere to, local policies.

Despite this, mobile phones fulfil a key purpose for students on placements. They enable you to contact your mentor and, as long as you keep your contact details up-to-date, they enable your mentor to contact you, or if your mentor is unwell, their colleagues can contact you easily. Tutors and mentors complain at length about the problem of students changing their mobile phone numbers without letting them know, so please have the professional courtesy to keep everyone up-to-date about your contact details.

Understand how to manage if you have a part-time job

Your first responsibility is to your education programme and attendance at your course and at your placements is of the highest importance. However, the funding that you receive to enable you to undertake the programme is limited, and for many students it is necessary to take on part-time work to supplement their income. There are different ways of managing to earn money, and there are also some constraints with regards to the type of work you take on.

Your part-time job mustn't compromise your ability to go in to university for the academic aspects of your programme, or you will find that you get behind on your work, or do not produce academic work at the standard you are capable of. This will be stressful for you, as work mounts up and you are under pressure to attend for teaching, as well as do the hours that you have agreed to do in your part-time job.

When you are in placements, ensuring that you turn up for work according to the duty rota must take precedence over the demands of your part-time job. You cannot say to the ward sister that you, for example, are unable to do late shifts because of your evening job in a pub or restaurant.

+..

Exercise 14.8

What examples can you think of where a part-time job could make it difficult for you to manage your placement hours? Why might this be the case?

....

Many students, if they have been healthcare assistants (HCAs) prior to commencing their nurse education programme, take on HCA work to earn extra money. There are some professional aspects of this that should be considered. If you are working as an HCA in the hospital where your placements are, then you should never work as an HCA on the same ward as your placement. This, if it happens, makes it harder for you to be a student, learning in practice, and causes your colleagues confusion, for, despite the likelihood that you will be in a different uniform (depending on whether you are an 'HCA' or a 'student') colleagues will not have time to consider these nuances as they organize work for the shift. Having different roles in the same ward will also cause your patients some difficulties, for they may ask you to help them with something that, as a student, you have not yet been assessed as competent to do for them, although you are able to perform similar tasks as an HCA. If you have been an HCA at that hospital, say on a medical elderly care ward, you may wish to not return to that ward as a student nurse. HCAs who do their nurse education programme say that if they go back to their former ward, everyone still sees them as an HCA, and they find it difficult to help their colleagues understand that they need to be treated as *students*, learning clinical and professional skills.

When students are worried about money, as is often the case, it is tempting to take on as much part-time work as possible. This has been discussed in Chapter 3. Try and consider what this might mean. From a professional perspective, arriving on placement for an early shift very tired after doing a late shift as an HCA will have an impact on how you cope in your placement. Even though you have high standards of professional behaviour, you won't be able to learn and, at an extreme level, you may compromise the safety of your patients because you are too exhausted to notice something important that has changed in one of your patients.

Understand why it is important to manage your time

This is about the 'time-management' aspect of professional behaviour, and learning to cope with the challenges posed by being a full-time student with a part-time job will be important in your successful completion of your course.

For an increasing number of students, who commence their nursing programme when they are older, rather than on leaving school or college, family concerns play a key part in managing time. Many prospective students, during their interviews for the programme, go into considerable detail about their childcare arrangements, and the support they have organized in their home life to enable them to take on what they realize will be a complex and demanding course. The mature approach that these students demonstrate suggests that they will have a good understanding of professional behaviour in the academic and practice settings.

Nevertheless, children do become unwell sometimes, and if a student has caring responsibilities towards others, such as older people, their best-laid plans for a smooth passage through placement may go off track. Making sure that, if they have to take time off to care for their family, they have let their placement know, and also let their mentor know, is still a professional approach to the situation. The same applies if the student is in the university, in terms of letting relevant tutors know.

This works for absences of 1 or 2 days, but if an absence is likely to be longer, the student must let their mentor and their personal tutor know how long they are likely to be away, and also discuss whether they will still be able to complete their placement hours in time, before moving on to the next stage of their programme. Staff and tutors will do their utmost to support a student who has a genuine problem, so it is best to be open about any issues that are causing you to miss your study or placement hours.

+ ···

Exercise 14.9

Imagine that you are a mentor. What would concern you if you didn't hear from a student who should be on duty? In what ways would their absence cause you stress or concern, in an already busy working situation? Think about two different students: Samantha, who until then has always arrived on time, ready to learn and is enthusiastic; and Marina, who has only been on time once in 2 weeks, never saying why she is late so often?

You can probably see that no situation is clear-cut, and that the professional approach is for each student to talk about anything that might affect his or her attendance at placement.

···

Understand the need for professional behaviour at university

When you are studying in the university setting, the people you are most likely to be working with are your peers, and your lecturers and teachers. There are a number of important things to remember about behaving as a professional in this setting. In teaching, and for fellow students, some individuals can have a noticeable impact on how teaching sessions work out through their understanding of how to behave in this environment. It is always much easier to learn in an organized and calm environment, whether this in a university teaching room or when you are working independently. The following scenario aims to show how personal behaviour and a lack of understanding of professional behaviour can affect a teaching session.

Incident

On Monday, the teaching session on heart disease was due to start at nine o'clock. The teaching room was on the ground floor in the main teaching block, and was easily reached from the bus stop and the car park where a few students had parked their cars. Out of a group of students, the majority had arrived slightly early, by eight forty-five, and were settled in their seats, waiting for the tutor to set up the presentation and organize the session materials. The tutor took a register at nine o'clock, and noticed that 10 people had not yet arrived. After asking the students if they knew of anyone who was off sick, he realized that 4 students were either going to be absent or late. As he started speaking, the door opened and 2 students came in laughing about something. They didn't greet the tutor, and sat down noisily in chairs halfway along a row, causing some disruption to other students who were writing notes. Ten minutes later, another student arrived, and finding that there were no available seats, pulled a chair off a stack and dumped it at the back. The tutor, who had stopped speaking while this was happening, started again. The session went on, until a student's mobile phone started ringing, using a loud ring-tone. The student fumbled in their bag on the floor, and eventually switched the tone off. The tutor reminded everyone that mobile phones must be switched off during teaching sessions. One student saw an amusing message on her phone as she was turning it off. She showed the message to her friend, and they laughed, causing other students to turn round. The tutor asked everyone to settle down, and be quiet. Looking around the group, he noticed that someone in the back row was indeed quiet, because they were asleep. When he then asked the students to move into small groups, he told the sleeping student to wake up, and then asked them why they had fallen asleep. The student replied that she had been out until four o'clock in the morning celebrating her friend's birthday, so was too tired. The tutor suggested that she go home as there was no point in her sleeping through the rest of the teaching session. He asked her to arrange an appointment with her personal tutor to discuss her behaviour. The rest of the session passed almost without incident, except for a drink spilling over the floor as the students moved out of their groups. This was despite a known policy about prohibiting students to bring drinks or food into classrooms and lecture theatres.

+ ....

Exercise 14.10

Think about how the students behaved in the teaching session. What is the impact of their various disruptions on their fellow students who had made the effort to arrive on time and be organized? What is the impact on their tutor? What could be the impact on the teaching session as a whole?

....

Although professional behaviour in clinical placements is rightly emphasized as of great importance, there is also a lot to think about with regards to behaving in a professional manner during the academic part of the education programme, at university.

14.4 Unprofessional behaviour and how to avoid it!

One student nurse said that it was 'almost useful' when a nurse or mentor she worked with showed what she felt was unprofessional behaviour. It demonstrated to her that she should not behave in the same way. She gave the example of when a mentor and student had been speaking to a patient about his admission to hospital. Afterwards, the mentor said 'I knew he would be difficult to talk to. He took forever to answer my questions'. The student felt that her mentor's behaviour was unprofessional, and that she expected the student to agree with her negative view of the patient, emphasizing her professional shortcomings to the student nurse.

Student comment

66 Keep the NMC Code in mind at all times. It will help you to assess whether nurses in practice are meeting the high standards of professional behaviour. Being shouted at by qualified staff, and in the presence of patients, is not professional behaviour. If this happens tell someone. 99

One of the most important aspects of professional behaviour for students is that their mentors, colleagues and tutors are knowledgeable and up-to-date in their theoretical and practical work. Students need to have reliable role models who can show them 'how it is done'.

So think about this as you complete your pre-registration programme. It is only the beginning of your learning, and your future responsibilities as a practising nurse, as a teacher of future students and as a role model, will always be of the utmost importance to you, your patients and clients and future colleagues.

Summary

This chapter has introduced what is meant by professional behaviour. It has done so by helping you to understand the reason why we directed you in earlier chapters to do, or not to do, some things. In time you will be able to make these links for yourself. There is a lot to think about as you develop the necessary professional behaviour to be successful. We suggest that key to this success is, from the moment you start on your pre-registration programme, to conduct yourself as the future professional and member of the nursing profession that you are.

■ Top tips

- Like theory and practice professional behaviour can be learned.
- Your appearance matters, especially in practice.
- If you want to be a registered nurse your behaviour in your personal life matters as much as your behaviour at university and in practice.
- Professional worries should always be shared. Do not go it alone.
- Always strive to practise to the highest standard.
- Use the resources at the NMC website and the online resource to keep up-to-date with changes.

■ Online resource centre

 For links to the student code of practice and other useful websites go to:
www.oxfordtextbooks.co.uk/orc/hart

■ References

Disability Discrimination Act (2005): http://www.direct.gov.uk/en/DisabledPeople/RightsAnd Obligations/DisabilityRight/DG_4001068

Nursing and Midwifery Council (2005): An NMC guide for students of nursing and midwifery: http://www.nmc-uk.org

Nursing and Midwifery Council (2008) The code: standards of conduct, performance and ethics for nurses and midwives: http://www.nmc-uk.org/aArticle.aspx?ArticleID=3056

Peach Report (1999) The Report of the UKCC Commission for Nursing and Midwifery Education, chaired by Sir Leonard Peach (UKCC, 1999).

Quality Assurance Agency (2001) *Content of curriculum and quality assurance*: www.qaa.ac.uk

Quality Assurance Agency (2002) *Content of curriculum and quality assurance:* www.qaa.ac.uk

■ Further reading

Criminal Records Bureau Home Page: http://www.crb.gov.uk

Department of Health (1998) Data Protection Act: http://www.opsi.gov.uk/Acts/Acts1998/ukpga_19980029_en_1

Fitness for Practice: http://www.nursingnetukcom/policies

Griffith R. and Tengnah C (2008) *Law, Ethics and Professional Issues in Nursing*. Transforming Nursing Practice: Common Foundation Programme. Learning Matters Ltd.

Mental Capacity Act (2005): http://www.opsi.gov.uk/ACTS/acts2005/ukpga_20050009_en_1

Moore D (2005) *Assuring Fitness for Practice: A Policy Review*. Nursing and Midwifery Council.

Nursing and Midwifery Council (2002) Practitioner–client relationships and the prevention of abuse: http://www.nmc-uk.org

Nursing and Midwifery Council (2004) Standards of Proficiency for Pre Registration Nursing Education: http://www.nmc-uk.org

Nursing and Midwifery Council (2005) Fitness to Practise: http://www.nmc-uk.org

Nursing and Midwifery Council (2005) Record Keeping Advice Sheet: http://www.nmc-uk.org

Nursing and Midwifery Council (2006) Gifts and Gratuities: http://www.nmc-uk.org

Nursing and Midwifery Council (2008) Consent: http://www.nmc-uk.org/aArticle.aspx?ArticleID=3056

Nursing and Midwifery Council (2008) Scenarios 1-3: Applying to University: http://www.nmc-uk.org/aArticle.aspx?ArticleID=3103

Nursing and Midwifery Council (2007) Guidance on Good Health and Good Character: http://www.nmc-uk.org/aArticle.aspx?ArticleID=2603

Nursing Times 29 April (2008) 104 (17): www.nursingtimes.net. The code: standards of conduct, performance and ethics for nurses and midwives.

Savage J and Moore L (2004) Interpreting accountability: an ethnographic study of practice nurses, accountability and multi-disciplinary team decision-making in the context of clinical governance. RCN Research Reports, London.

Schober J and Ash C (2005) *Student nurses' guide to professional practice and development*. Hodder Education, London.

Cracking the NMC code

Sheila Muller

The aims of this chapter are:

➤ To help you to understand the meaning of The Code (NMC 2008) for registered nurses

➤ To assist in the development of your own professional behaviour

➤ To help you to recognize when others may not be acting professionally

Once you have completed the pre-registration programme, registered as a nurse and taken up your first post, you will be expected to work according to the guidelines in The Code. The following is an in-depth discussion of each of the statements in The Code with examples from practice. We have done this to help you understand how it works and how it links to your work as a nurse. Chapter 14 made reference to what happens when a nurse's conduct falls short of what is required. A sure way of avoiding such difficulties in the future and to develop your understanding of professional behaviour is to know The Code inside out.

Nurse teacher comment

❝ You should have been given a copy of The Code by your teachers. It is important that you have one. And read it. It can also be accessed at the NMC website: **www. nmc-uk.org.** ❞

As you read, you will start to see how The Code has an impact on you and your patients and clients, while you are looking after them. It will also become clear that how you conduct yourself in your personal life (even miles away from the university and clinical practice) is also very important. Your personal behaviour 'acting lawfully' and upholding 'the reputation of your profession' affects how others perceive you as a professional nurse and the nursing profession as a whole.

In reality, you are unlikely to think about The Code consciously every minute of your day. Your mind will be occupied by the activity of the moment. That is why it is important that you read and re-read this chapter, so that the messages become second nature to you. Professional behaviour guides everything you do as a registered nurse. Do not worry; you have 3 years to develop this and that learning starts now.

Student comment

66 Don't let the words 'standards of conduct' put you off reading the NMC code. It is easy and simple to use in practice and will help you a lot to be a good nurse. 99

15.1 **Standards of conduct, performance and ethics for nurses and midwives**

What follows is a page by page discussion of The Code. For clarity blue represent sections of the code.

The NMC Code The people in your care must be able to trust you with their health and well-being.

To justify that trust, you must:

- Make the care of people your first concern, treating them as individuals and respecting their dignity.
- Work with others to protect and promote the health and well-being of those in your care, their families and carers, and the wider community.
- Provide a high standard of practice and care at all times.
- Be open and honest, act with integrity and uphold the reputation of your profession.

As a professional, you are personally accountable for actions and omissions in your practice and must always be able to justify your decisions.

You must always act lawfully, whether those laws relate to your professional practice or personal life.

Failure to comply with this Code of Conduct may bring your fitness to practise into question and endanger your registration.

This Code of Conduct should be considered together with the Nursing and Midwifery Council's rules, standards, guidance and advice available from **www.nmc-uk.org**

Exercise 15.1

Look again at the section above and pick out some key words and phrases. You might choose 'trust' or 'integrity'. Get a sheet of paper and write out what each of these means to you as you think about nursing. For some of you, it might have been a personal experience of being a patient, cared for by a nurse. For others it might be about realizing that a patient completely trusted you as you looked after them. You could also think about whether there have been occasions when a patient has experienced fear or anxiety because they have not felt able to trust the nurses or other health professionals who are looking after them.

The NMC Code Make the care of people your first concern, treating them as individuals and respecting their dignity.

Treat people as individuals:

- You must treat people as individuals and respect their dignity.
- You must not discriminate in any way against those in your care.
- You must treat people kindly and considerately.
- You must act as an advocate for those in your care, helping them to access relevant health and social care, information and support.

Can you remember occasions when you have not been treated as an individual, or felt that you have not been treated with respect? Perhaps this was when you were at school, or if you were travelling from place to place, or in a crowd.

Exercise 15.2

Now think about how it feels to be sick and in hospital, vulnerable to everything that happens to you. You may have had experience of being a patient and can think about how this felt for you at the time. If you have never been in hospital ask people you know about their experiences.

Make notes about what you think would be most important to a patient, in being cared for.

When talking with people who have had experience of being patients, they can too often give an example of feeling that they were not being treated as an individual, or with dignity. They always remember these occasions, because they felt so upset. Read through the examples below and think about how you would do things differently, to protect people's individuality and dignity.

+ ···

Nursing practice example 1

Mr Richards, a gentleman in his seventies, was admitted 2 days ago to a mental health unit, with acute anxiety. When the nurse was admitting him, she asked about his food preferences. He said that he was unable to eat cheese as it upset his stomach. When the lunch arrived on the ward Mr Richards was given a plate of macaroni cheese. Nobody asked if that was the right meal for him. Mr Richards didn't eat the lunch; he just stared at the plate wondering what to do. The nurse did not comment on why he had not eaten anything, she just took the plate away. She assumed (incorrectly) that he just didn't want to eat. He wasn't treated as an individual, with needs; he was not cared for. He was hungry.

Nursing practice example 2

Mrs Thompson had been pressing her buzzer for ten minutes. She needed to use a commode, and wasn't able to walk out to the bathroom. A nurse arrived, asked what she wanted and fetched the commode. The nurse was in a hurry, so after sitting Mrs Thompson on the commode she rushed off, leaving the curtains open, so that anyone walking past could see her sitting there. She couldn't get up and close the curtains herself, so she had to endure sitting there, feeling extremely vulnerable, her personal dignity in shreds. She was there for 20 minutes, as nobody came back to see if she was all right.

Nursing practice example 3

Jane has a severe learning disability and needs help with all aspects of her personal care, including needing support to eat. Sitting in her chair after lunch, the remains of food she has not swallowed are forming a red stain down the front of her jumper. The healthcare assistant forgot to give her a drink after lunch as agreed in her care plan.

+ ···

Exercise 15.3 Consider the following for the three nursing practice examples above:

- How do you think each of those people felt?
- Think about Jane, who may have not been aware of how she looked. Does this matter?
- List all of the things that fell below professional standards of care.
- How would you prevent them happening to people in your care?

Something that people who have been patients, particularly older people, often comment on is that nurses, having found out their first names, call them by these names, rather than using Mr or Mrs and their surname. Nurses and other health professionals should always find out how each individual wishes to be addressed, and not make assumptions. Some nurses call everyone 'darling' or 'love', which means that they do not see each person as an individual.

The NMC Code Make the care of people your first concern, treating them as individuals and respecting their dignity.

Respect people's confidentiality:

- You must respect people's right to confidentiality.
- You must ensure people are informed about how and why information is shared by those who will be providing their care.
- You must disclose information if you believe someone may be at risk of harm, in line with the law of the country in which you are practising.

Each individual has the right to expect that information held about them is accurate and up-to-date. A cornerstone of confidentiality is the Data Protection Act (1998), which is a key piece of legislation that affects you personally and professionally, and you must be aware of what you must do to comply with it. The overall aim of the Data Protection Act is that it gives rights to individuals about the personal information held about them. Personal data is information about a living individual who can be identified from the information, and it encompasses both facts and opinions about each individual.

As a professional nurse, or nursing student, if you process (i.e. collect, use, disclose or keep) any personal data about people, you must play your part in making sure that you respect their data protection rights, with regard to written and electronic records. For example, your placement area may be asked to supply copies of the personal data you hold about a patient, and the placement area must be able to do this. The Data Protection Act protects these rights.

Any personal data must be reviewed regularly making sure it is kept up-to-date, kept securely and deleted when it is no longer required. Somebody in each ward or community team is the contact and takes responsibility for every set of personal data that is held.

As a student nurse, you will *not* have responsibility for ensuring that all records held about patients in the placement area comply with the Data Protection Act. However, you will be asked to write in patient records, record personal information (e.g. when admitting a patient to a ward), and are quite likely to find yourself being asked about patients by relatives or friends. All patient records are legal documents, and, in the rare occurrence of being part of a court case, can be included as evidence, perhaps of something that was done, but instead as evidence that something was not done, and the patient suffered as a result.

As we have stressed in previous chapters, never be tempted to take on responsibility that exceeds your student status. An example of this might be that a relative asks you about how a patient is, or what illness he or she has. You should refer the relative to the person in charge, explaining that, as a student, you cannot give any information. If a patient wishes to speak to you in confidence, you should also explain that they should speak to someone else, the senior nurse or your mentor, rather than leaving you to take responsibility that exceeds your role as a student.

The NMC Code Make the care of people your first concern, treating them as individuals and respecting their dignity.

Collaborate with those in your care:

- You must listen to the people in your care and respond to their concerns and preferences.
- You must support people in caring for themselves to improve and maintain their health.
- You must recognise and respect the contribution that people make to their own care and wellbeing.
- You must make arrangements to meet people's language and communication needs.
- You must share with people, in a way they can understand, the information they want or need to know about their health.

On your pre-registration programme, you will learn about how to communicate with patients and clients. Some students have said that when they listen to colleagues communicate with people, asking questions, giving information and talking at the patient's level, they feel that they aspire to be like that nurse. On the other hand, a nurse who is impatient, giving lists of instructions or talking 'at' a patient, is not a good role model. One of the most important skills is listening to others, who may be feeling very unwell or in considerable pain. They may have English as a second language and find it difficult to let people know what they need, or perhaps what is causing them to worry or be anxious. As a student looking after people, you have a wonderful opportunity to give them your full attention, responding to their concerns and ensuring that you also communicate clearly and accurately to qualified staff any concerns that patients and clients have expressed to you.

The NMC Code Make the care of people your first concern, treating them as individuals and respecting their dignity.

Ensure you gain consent:

- You must ensure that you gain consent before you begin any treatment or care.
- You must respect and support people's rights to accept or decline treatment and care.
- You must uphold people's rights to be fully involved in decisions about their care.
- You must be aware of the legislation regarding mental capacity, ensuring that people who lack capacity remain at the centre of decision making and are fully safeguarded.
- You must be able to demonstrate that you have acted in someone's best interests if you have provided care in an emergency.

This applies to all individuals, and ensures that when they are told about proposed treatment or care, that the information is given to them in a sensitive way, to enable them to understand what is proposed, and have enough time to consider the information and ask questions. People also need enough information to help them make their decision, and exercise their right to accept or decline the treatment or procedure that has been discussed. Each adult is presumed to have the mental capacity (Mental Capacity Act 2005) to consent to or refuse treatment, unless they are unable to take in or understand the information provided, or unable to use the information provided in making their decision. An exception to this is in an emergency situation, where an adult who is not able to consent, perhaps because they are unconscious, may have the treatment necessary to preserve their life (see Chapter 16 for more about this).

The NMC Code Make the care of people your first concern, treating them as individuals and respecting their dignity.

Maintain clear professional boundaries:

- You must refuse any gifts, favours or hospitality that might be interpreted as an attempt to gain preferential treatment.
- You must not ask for or accept loans from anyone in your care or anyone close to them.
- You must establish and actively maintain clear sexual boundaries at all times with people in your care, their families and carers.

When the people you have looked after want to express their gratitude for your care, they may offer you gifts, favours or hospitality. The Code is clear in stating that if this might be interpreted as an attempt to gain preferential treatment, and the offer must be refused. If you are unsure about what to do, then you should speak to your mentor or tutor, and they can guide you about the local policies that can clarify the situation.

An important part of portraying correct professional behaviour is that good relationships with your patients and clients require warmth and empathy on the part of the professional. Also, friendships and professional healthcare relationships do have some similarities, but there are a number of important differences. See Chapter 16 for more about emotional and sexual boundaries.

The NMC Code Work with others to protect and promote the health and wellbeing of those in your care, their families and carers, and the wider community.

Share information with your colleagues:

- You must keep your colleagues informed when you are sharing the care of others.
- You must work with colleagues to monitor the quality of your work and maintain the safety of those in your care.
- You must facilitate students and others to develop their competence.

Nursing is a collaborative profession, and the best outcomes for patients and clients are achieved when staff work together effectively. As a student, one of your responsibilities is to make sure that others are aware of the care you are giving. You will be working with qualified staff, healthcare assistants and other students, and all have a shared responsibility to ensure that your patients and clients are safe, and their care is of the best quality.

The NMC Code Work with others to protect and promote the health and wellbeing of those in your care, their families and carers, and the wider community.

Work effectively as part of a team:

* You must work cooperatively within teams and respect the skills, expertise and contributions of your colleagues.
* You must be willing to share your skills and experience for the benefit of your colleagues.
* You must consult and take advice from colleagues, when appropriate.
* You must treat your colleagues fairly and without discrimination.
* You must make a referral to another practitioner when it is in the best interests of someone in your care.

As Chapters 10 and 11 have highlighted, working as a team is essential in delivering high-quality care to your patients and clients. It also helps in managing the workload that is expected of all health professionals. As a student, you will be assisting with care, and only as a senior student will you have a greater share of caring responsibilities. So your role is concerned with supporting your colleagues, helping them and learning through what you are doing.

Equality means that each person in that team must be treated equally, valuing each person's participation and contribution, and ensuring that they have the opportunity to fulfil their potential. It also clearly applies to each patient and client in your care. Diversity focuses on the understanding, respect and valuing of all physical, cultural and social differences among individuals, and applies to all the people you care for, and your colleagues. See Chapter 16 for more about working well with patient and clients.

The NMC Code Work with others to protect and promote the health and wellbeing of those in your care, their families and carers, and the wider community.

Delegate effectively:

* You must establish that anyone you delegate to is able to carry out your instructions.
* You must confirm that the outcome of any delegated task meets required standards.
* You must make sure that everyone you are responsible for is supervised and supported.

As a student it is *you* who are most likely to be the person who is delegated to by registered staff. As a junior student, you must always be supervised in carrying out any procedures, treatment or tasks. As a senior student you need to feel confident that you can carry out any delegated instructions safely and competently, and feel able to speak up if you, perhaps, have not done a procedure before, or have little experience.

+··

Exercise 15.4

Think about how senior staff delegate to you. Notice when they do it skilfully; notice when you feel *instructed*. Why do you enjoy working with some staff more than others? Is it because they value your contribution? How will you delegate when you are a registered nurse?

··

The NMC Code Work with others to protect and promote the health and wellbeing of those in your care, their families and carers, and the wider community.

Manage risk:

- You must act without delay if you believe that you, a colleague or anyone else may be putting someone at risk.
- You must inform someone in authority if you experience problems that prevent you working within this Code or other nationally agreed standards.
- You must report your concerns in writing if problems in the environment of care are putting people at risk.

The management of risk is very important, and applies not only to the treatment given to patients and clients, but also to the care environment. There is an emphasis on anticipating and preventing risk, rather than reacting to a proven risk. It may be, for example, that the area where you are on placement is untidy, with equipment left out, causing a fire or trip hazard. Another example might be where a patient cannot reach for water or tissues without the risk of falling out of bed.

Nursing practice example 4 describes a situation where a patient was put at risk. Write out some ways of minimizing the risks.

+··

Nursing practice example 4

Karen had undergone surgery to her back four days earlier. The operation had gone well and she was feeling well. She decided to go for a walk along the ward to the bathroom at the other end of the ward, wearing a long nightgown and no slippers, as they had been left out of reach under her bed. The journey to and from the bathroom was achieved without incident and, as she was climbing back into bed, the ward sister came up to speak with her.

What risks could you list? As a start, you might think that her long nightgown might have caused her to trip...

··

List of potential risks:

Another risk that you may not have thought of: Karen should have stayed in bed, as her back surgery meant that she should not have been walking around at all!

The NMC Code Provide a high standard of practice and care at all times.

Use the best available evidence:

- You must deliver care based on the best available evidence or best practice.
- You must ensure any advice you give is evidence based, if you are suggesting healthcare products or services.
- You must ensure that the use of complementary or alternative therapies is safe and in the best interests of those in your care.

As a student, working under supervision, you will not be in the position of deciding on the care that is to be delivered. However, as a learner, your own academic studies and previous experience in placements should be ensuring that you are developing your understanding of evidence based practice. The principle of evidence based practice is that clinical decisions should be based on the best available evidence, usually derived from research at an international, national or local level. It emphasizes the importance of consulting well-conducted systematic research to inform clinical decisions. Increasingly, patients research their own information about healthcare products and services, and complementary or alternative therapies. They may well talk to you about what they have found out, perhaps to check on whether their information is correct. So, the greater your own knowledge about the evidence base for treatments, medicines and products, the more you can ensure that patients have accurate knowledge.

If you do, however, feel that a patient is advocating alternatives that have no proven benefits, it would be a good idea to discuss the situation with a registered nurse or your mentor.

The NMC Code Provide a high standard of practice and care at all times.

Keep your skills and knowledge up to date:

- You must have the knowledge and skills for safe and effective practice when working without direct supervision.
- You must recognise and work within the limits of your competence.
- You must keep your knowledge and skills up to date throughout your working life.
- You must take part in appropriate learning and practice activities that maintain and develop your competence and performance.

As you go through your pre-registration programme you will always be a learner, and your responsibility, and the responsibility of your teachers and mentors, is to ensure that you develop up-to-date knowledge and skills, so that from being a junior student up to qualifying and beyond, you are able to practise safely and effectively as a professional. As a junior student you will be working with direct supervision, but as a more senior student and then after you qualify, you won't have direct supervision, so it will be up to you to continue to practise safely.

The next point in the box above gives another perspective on your knowledge and skills. It focuses on all professionals in that they must understand the limits of their competence, so if they do not know what to do, or are unsure in any way, they ask for a competent person to carry out a piece of work, e.g. a clinical procedure. They may, however, decide that they will carry out the procedure but will ask for somebody who is competent to supervise them.

This is important for you as a student. You may feel that you *should* know how to do something. Perhaps your mentor makes the assumption that you know how to do a procedure. What do you do? Do you try and bluff your way through, hoping that nothing will go wrong?

Exercise 15.5

Think about a situation where you are the patient. A student nurse arrives to let you know that they want to change a complicated dressing, or remove a tube that has been draining from an infected site on your stomach. They seem nervous and unsure about how to do the task. How would you feel in those circumstances? Would you feel less anxious and more comfortable if that student asked for someone to observe and instruct them, or if they asked a qualified nurse to show them what to do?

Looking at it from the perspective of your patient or client, they will be much less anxious when they know that those looking after them are fully knowledgeable and competent.

The NMC Code Provide a high standard of practice and care at all times.

Keep clear and accurate records:

- You must keep clear and accurate records of the discussions you have, the assessments you make, the treatment and medicines you give and how effective these have been.
- You must complete records as soon as possible after an event has occurred.
- You must not tamper with original records in any way.
- You must ensure any entries you make in someone's paper records are clearly and legibly signed, dated and timed.
- You must ensure any entries you make in someone's electronic records are clearly attributable to you.
- You must ensure all records are kept securely.

You will be taught about the importance of accurate documentation and record-keeping. Each NHS Trust, and other services you may be placed in, will have an agreed policy about the writing, storage and maintenance of written and electronic documentation about the care given to each person. It is one of the most important things to get right in your practice, and learning to complete records and documents to the highest standard will help protect your patients, and will also protect you, should there ever be any question about a patient you have looked after.

Members of the public have the right to expect that healthcare professionals will practice a high standard of record-keeping. The quality of a professional's record-keeping is a reflection of the standard of their professional practice. Good record-keeping is a mark of a skilled and safe practitioner, while careless or incomplete record-keeping often highlights wider problems with someone's practice. For more about record-keeping, see the online resource.

Some of the most important considerations with regard to record-keeping and documentation are the legal aspects that all nurses, students and qualified staff should be aware of. The legal aspects of the completion and management of records applies to manual (written) and electronic records. However, although there are some agreed standards, there will be differences between NHS Trusts, and between all the professional groups in the NHS in terms of content, format and local standards, so when you are on clinical placement, it is very important that you understand local policies for the documentation of care, and adhere to these.

As a student, everything you do for a patient can be written down in patients' care plans, but must also be countersigned by your mentor or a qualified member of the nursing staff. Although you are responsible for what you do, and what you write, ultimately the qualified staff is accountable legally and to the NMC for the care that you give.

+ ....

Exercise 15.6

When you go into a new placement, take the time to look closely at patients' or clients' records. Read what the each member of staff has written, and also note that each record of care has the date written clearly and has been signed by the person who gave that care. Think about whether the records are, as is required, written neatly, legibly and in black ink.

....

Although the vast majority of health professionals do their best to keep records of a high standard, occasionally a case emerges where this is not the case, either because of poor practice, or (very rarely) through deliberate actions.

Record-keeping and the protection of individual patients, came into the spotlight a few years ago, when a GP, Dr Harold Shipman was convicted of the deaths of a number of his patients. Most of the people who died were older women, many of them over 75 years old, who died soon after he had given them a lethal dose of a medication. The outcomes of the investigation indicated, among other things, that his standard of record-keeping was poor, and it was not possible to make an accurate assessment of the content of the records. Nevertheless, one finding was that some records contained back dated entries, making it impossible for investigators to reach any conclusions about what had happened to each of those people at the time. Following this case, recommendations included regularly review- ing general practice records, and the recording of information about medication that has been given to patients.

Maintaining clear and accurate records is a time-consuming task for everyone and wher- ever you are on placement, this work must be completed.

Exercise 15.7 Consider what might be some of the implications for a patient if the nurse does not complete the documentation properly.

Some suggestions are:

If there is missing data on observations, such as blood pressure measurements, then a nurse or doctor, who is reviewing that patient's condition, would be unable to make an accurate assessment about any changes.

If a nurse on night duty, who is trying to learn about a patient's progress, cannot read the records because they are written illegibly, then they might miss something important. For example, the notes may document that a dose of Ibuprofen was given orally in the morning to ease post-operative pain, but the next sentence is illegible, so the night nurse doesn't know that the patient felt unwell after this and vomited, so may be intolerant to Ibuprofen. She might then give the patient another dose, causing a risk to the patient.

Try and think of an example of your own, or map out some of the possible implications for a patient if there are mistakes in their records.

Sally Jackson is a first-year student on a busy ward children's ward. She is helping to look after three patients under the supervision of her mentor. The mentor is called away to help another member of staff. Sally is completing record sheets that document how much each child has been drinking throughout the day. As she completes the sheet for one child she realizes that she might have forgotten to put in some readings from his drinks earlier in the day. She is worried that her mentor will tell her off for forgetting, so she quickly writes in two sets of numbers, 100 ml and 150 ml, indicating to anyone else reading the sheet that the child has had two drinks. Except he hasn't! He has been feeling quite unwell throughout the morning, and has been rather sleepy. The mentor returns and checks all the sheets, and believes the child is well hydrated and has been drinking well.

Exercise 15.8

What would be the potential impact of the altered records on the child?

What would be the impact on Sally Jackson, and the implications for her?

All patient records, written and electronic, must aim to comply with each NHS Trust's Information Governance and the NHS Litigation Authority Standards. NHS Trusts work to ensure that there are standards in place to ensure that this compliance is achieved. There has been considerable growth over recent years in the number of staff whose work focuses on investigating claims of clinical negligence, as people and families who may have been affected contact lawyers in order to claim compensation if an error in treatment or care has occurred.

So, protection of your patients is the most important aspect of ensuring excellent standards of record-keeping. The others who should be protected are staff, you and your colleagues from the health professions, who rely on each other's professionalism to protect yourselves from litigation. The annual cost to the NHS of legal claims from individuals and their families stands at over £90 million, and it increases every year.

The writing and keeping of accurate records is of immense importance in caring for people. Everyone knows people who write illegibly, who give you eyestrain as you try to work out each word. For patients and clients it is crucial that everything that concerns their care is documented clearly, and with accuracy.

A short case study provides some insight into why record-keeping is so important.

+ ....

Nursing practice example 5

Mrs Lewis has told the nurse that the medication she has been given for pain control after major surgery is not making any difference to her pain. She is tense and doesn't like to move around because it hurts to do so. The nurse asks the junior doctor to speak to Mrs Lewis, and after he has done so he decides to write a prescription for stronger medication. The night nurses arrive, and while they are doing their rounds Mrs Lewis asks for 'some of the new medicine' so that she can get some pain-free sleep. The night nurse looks at the medication sheet. She can just make out the name of the medication, but cannot read the dose that has been prescribed. Therefore she cannot give the medication, and time has to be spent by another doctor writing a prescription legibly. Meanwhile Mrs Lewis can't sleep as the pain is worse.

....

This is only one example of poor documentation. Others may involve writing up notes on a patient's care, or writing a form about something that has happened to a patient or client, e.g. if they fell over while walking or slipped while getting out of bed.

From a legal perspective, if something is not written down it 'didn't happen', so if there was litigation or a court case, accurate, clear and detailed documentation will enable lawyers to reach a full understanding of an event, and may well also protect the reputation of staff who were caring for someone. It is also important to write down an account of an event as soon as possible afterwards, because the longer you leave it, the less accurate it will be.

The NMC Code Be open and honest, act with integrity and uphold the reputation of your profession.

Act with integrity:

- You must demonstrate a personal and professional commitment to equality and diversity.
- You must adhere to the laws of the country in which you are practising.
- You must inform the NMC if you have been cautioned, charged or found guilty of a criminal offence.
- You must inform any employers you work for if your fitness to practise is impaired or is called into question.

As we saw earlier in Chapter 14, good character is fundamental to being a nurse or midwife. You must be honest and trustworthy in your behaviour and attitude to those you are caring for and your colleagues.

Although detailed checks are carried out before you start, on rare occasions during a student's pre-registration course something happens that causes them to be cautioned, charged or found guilty of a criminal offence. This might, for example, be a motoring offence. You must let your tutors know about any such event, and the NMC also needs to know. Depending on the nature of the event, you may still be allowed to continue as a student. Not letting your tutor know is likely to make any later disclosure of an offence much worse.

The NMC Code Be open and honest, act with integrity and uphold the reputation of your profession.

Deal with problems:

- You must give a constructive and honest response to anyone who complains about the care they have received.
- You must not allow someone's complaint to prejudice the care you provide for them.
- You must act immediately to put matters right if someone in your care has suffered harm for any reason.
- You must explain fully and promptly to the person affected what has happened and the likely effects.
- You must cooperate with internal and external investigations.

As a student, you will not have to address any of the above issues on your own. However, you do have a responsibility to let your qualified colleagues know if anyone in your care has suffered any potential harm, or if you have any concerns about their care. You could talk to your mentor, but if you feel that this is not possible, speak to the ward manager, or your personal tutor.

The NMC Code Be open and honest, act with integrity and uphold the reputation of your profession.

Be impartial:

- You must not abuse your privileged position for your own ends.
- You must ensure that your professional judgement is not influenced by any commercial considerations.

As a student, then as a registered nurse, you are required to maintain personal and professional integrity for yourself, for the profession and for the public. For some registered nurses, their work requires them to use commercially available products (e.g. nicotine-replacement products in smoking-cessation clinics). Nurses may be asked by companies to use one product in preference to another. The nurses' decision must be based entirely on clinical judgements.

Finally, when you become a registered nurse it is important always to uphold the reputation of the profession as follows:

The NMC Code Be open and honest, act with integrity and uphold the reputation of your profession.

Uphold the reputation of your profession:

- You must not use your professional status to promote causes that are not related to health.
- You must cooperate with the media only when you can confidently protect the confidential information and dignity of those in your care.
- You must uphold the reputation of your profession at all times.

Mentor comment

❝ It will help your success to remember that being a nursing student is different to the usual student experience, that you will be expected to be professional, comply with a code of conduct and that you have to achieve the necessary standards both practically and academically. ❞

Summary

By now you should be feeling more comfortable with The Code and what it expects of registered nurses. You are advised to return again and again to this chapter and Chapter 14 until you feel confident that you understand the professional behaviour required of you. There are many more examples we could have given. For each section, work out some for yourself. This will aid you learning and help your success.

■ Top tips

- ■ The Code is designed to support nurses in their practice.
- ■ Read it and know it and the implications of it, inside out.
- ■ Be safe.

■ Online resource centre

 We strongly advise that you find out more about equality and diversity in the work place. You can do this by following the link at: **www.oxfordtextbooks.co.uk/orc/hart/**

■ References

Data Protection Act (1998): **www.opsi.gov.uk/Acts/Acts1998/ukpga_19980029_en_1**

Mental Capacity Act (2005): **www.opsi.gov.uk/acts/acts2005/ukpga_20050009_en_1**

NHS Litigation Authority Standards. **http://www.nhsla.com/home**

Nursing and Midwifery Council (2008) *The code: standards of conduct, performance and ethics for nurses and midwives:* **http://www.nmc-uk.org/aArticle.aspx?ArticleID=3056**

The Shipman Reports 2002–05: **http://www.the-shipman-inquiry.org.uk/reports.asp**

■ Further reading

Tschudin V (ed.) (2003) *Approaches to ethics; nursing beyond boundaries.* Butterworth Heinemann, Oxford.

PART 3

Thriving and surviving

Challenges you may face

Sue Hart

The aims of this chapter are:

➤ To raise awareness about some of the challenges you may face

➤ To offer practical suggestions and advice about how to deal with these

➤ To guide you regarding emotional and sexual boundaries with patients

➤ To help you to understand what happens when a patient dies

This chapter looks at some of the areas that we know students can find difficult. How you react to situations, communicate and work with people who have different needs, says a lot about your potential as a future registered nurse. Your success in clinical practice will be enhanced by working well with your mentor. Most of the time the student–mentor relationship works well on both sides. But what if it does not?

16.1 Problems with your mentor? Some ways to put it right

Student comment

❝ On my second placement I learnt something really important. I did not like the nurse who was my mentor. I thought he was sarcastic at times; he thought he was funny. When I talked to my personal tutor she asked if I was getting opportunities to meet my outcomes. I had done everything I needed and he had done everything he should. It was just a personality clash. I realized I just had to get on with it. ❞

If you do not get along with your mentor and *this is affecting your learning*, you need to do something, as doing nothing may risk your ability to achieve the outcomes. Do not pretend that everything is fine. You could talk about this to your personal tutor or the link tutor. Alternatively, the best option may be to discuss the situation directly with your mentor or the nurse in charge. As an adult learner you are responsible for your own learning; as a registered nurse you may often have to handle potentially difficult situations.

The following are suggestions for opening such a conversation with your mentor.

I feel concerned I am not really learning enough from you in this placement, is there something we could do about this?

I'm worried that there may be something between us which is having an impact on my learning; could we talk it over please?

Remember, you have a limited time in clinical practice so you must really make the most of it and learn all you can.

What if your mentor insists you do something and you do not feel confident?

The registered practitioners are responsible for the consequences of the actions and omissions of a student in placement. If your mentor asks you to do something without assessing whether you are capable, and something should go wrong, it is the mentor that takes responsibility and is accountable. However, you also have some responsibility here. If you are asked to do something that you feel you are not capable of, then it is regarded as your responsibility to tell your mentor this before you attempt the task.

Nancy, I need to tell you that I have not yet done XYZ on my own, and do not feel competent. May I observe you first please?

 See the latest NMC student guidelines at the online resource about working with your mentor.

What if I you think your mentor has done something wrong?

There may be times when you are unsure about why your mentor is doing something. There may also be times when you think that your mentor is doing something wrong. Students are well-placed to question why something is or is not being done. If you feel your mentor is doing something wrong, you must act, even though this may feel difficult. You may be observing misconduct. If your mentor is unable to provide you with a satisfactory explanation, talk to the person in charge, your personal teacher or use the advisory service provided by the NMC. Be confident that the NMC supports the questioning of registered practitioners. The safety of the public is paramount.

✛ ....

Exercise 16.1

Search the term 'whistle blowing' on the NMC website. The term means to inform on a nurse who is doing something they should not. At the time of writing the NMC are developing practical guidelines to support this activity.

....

Nurse teacher comment

❝ Not all practice that you observe will be exemplary, but whilst not constituting misconduct, it might be less than perfect. Make yourself a promise that you will not perpetuate such practice and will not be repeating what you have observed. ❞

16.2 **What if a complaint is made about you?**

As Chapter 9 noted, it is possible to learn a lot from situations where a complaint has been made. But what if the complaint is made about you?

Occasionally, patients and clients do make complaints about the care they receive from students. This can be for a variety of reasons, including simple misunderstandings. It is important to make sure that you are aware of the local procedures for dealing with complaints. If a patient indicates *to you* that they are unhappy about their treatment or care, you should report the matter immediately to your mentor. Alternatively, a complaint *about you* might be made to your mentor or another registered nurse. Your mentor will then need to speak with the person directly about their complaint.

What happens now depends on the circumstances. If the issue was that you said you would support the person to have a bath that afternoon and, they waited and you never came, a full and sincere apology may satisfy the complainant. A framework for this is simply to:

- Acknowledge your part in what happened.

- Explain why it happened.

- Show how you know it will not happen again.

- Apologize sincerely, as though you mean it.

Reflection can help following such situations, as below. Despite being motivated by the best intentions the student ran into difficulties.

Student comment

"I write down mistakes that I make in an attempt to learn from them; someone once told me it was a useful thing to do. The other day I answered a bell that had been ringing for a long time but was not on the side of the ward where I was working. There was a lady on a commode who wanted to get dressed. As it is a rehabilitation ward where people are encouraged to be as independent as possible, I got out her clothes, put them next to her on the bed, told her to do as much as she could herself and said that I would tell the nurse in charge of that side that she was ready to be helped. I then passed on the message to an HCA working with the nurse. This lady fell from the commode trying to get dressed and I heard the nurse telling her off for not ringing her bell. It was an awful feeling that I had intervened to try and help and ended up being partly responsible for her fall. I owned up to the nurse after things had been sorted out and apologized for getting involved. The HCA didn't say anything! I sensed that the nurse was really annoyed with me but sometimes you just have to take responsibility for your mistakes and admit that in trying to do your best sometimes things don't always work out. My mentor was really lovely and told me that it was not my fault that this lady had fallen and tried her hardest to reassure me. My learning from this was not to answer nurse calls in the morning in areas of the ward that I'm not working in, unless I have the time to commit to fully sorting out what is going on."

In more serious circumstances even a sincere apology is not sufficient. A student would most likely be withdrawn from the placement while an investigation takes place, involving both practice and the university. In such a scenario, the student is told what is happening and is kept informed regarding the findings and outcomes. If required to appear before the university fitness for practise panel (see Chapter 13), a student representative, friend or union representative can support the individual. Complaints can result in disciplinary action and removal from the course.

16.3 Working positively with all patients and clients: ensuring anti-discriminatory practice

As a registered nurse you will have a duty of care to all patients and clients irrespective of their *social, ethnic, cultural or religious background, their age, gender or sexual orientation and regardless* of any *disability physical, sensory, psychological or learning* that they may have. The term 'anti-discriminatory practice' (ADP) is often used in social and healthcare settings to describe this need for positive working and to be aware of one's own *values and beliefs* with regard to 'difference'. Also it is important to understand how cultural traditions may affect an individual's behaviour when ill.

ADP challenges professionals to reflect on their own practise and to address behaviour that could be regarded as oppressive, harsh and authoritarian or stigmatizing, and not seeing beyond a negative view of the person (Thompson 2006).

Some examples of discriminating behaviour

- Use of language that discriminates or stigmatizes.
- Withholding or delaying a service (including care by a nurse on a ward).
- Advantaging one group or one patient over another or others.
- Making judgements about individuals based on hearsay or your own prejudices.

+ ....

Exercise 16.2 Please read the following scenarios and consider if you believe the behaviour is discriminatory and, if so, how?

The operating department at your hospital has a monthly list of patients with learning disabilities who have dental work done under general anaesthetic, as they are unable to go to the dentist in the usual way. They are known as the '*mental dentals*'.

You hear:
    'Let's leave that gay one in the bed in the corner to last and hope he may have done his own wash when we get there.'

Or:
    'The trouble with Asian patients is the smell of that awful food they eat, makes me feel ill.'
    It could be argued that discrimination is taking place in all these examples. In order, there are disablist attitudes, homophobia and racism.

....

Exercise 16.3

Think back to before you started the course. You imagined yourself nursing patients and clients. Can you remember *now* who the patients in your imagination were?

....

By now you will have realized that patients and clients do not fall neatly into the NMC's four fields of practice. Irrespective of your future practice area, it is important that you show your mentors and teachers that you are able to work with *all* patients and clients who come into your care.

Cultural differences

People from minority ethnic groups may belong to one of many different religions. The 2001 census recorded that in the UK there are 42 million Christians; 1.6 million Muslims; 559,000 Hindus; 336,000 Sikhs; 267,000 Jews. The cultural beliefs and values of these groups vary and all healthcare professionals must be culturally sensitive to their particular needs. For example:

- It is against the belief of devout Jehovah's Witnesses to accept blood from another person, and they may refuse even if a condition is life threatening.

- Islam teaches modesty with regards to nakedness. Some Muslims may be distressed being cared for by a nurse of the opposite sex.

- Jewish people believe that there is life after death. It is important to an orthodox Jewish patient near the end of life to be seen by a Rabbi.

(For further reading see: Holland and Hogg 2001.)

Racism

People who hold racist views believe that all members of a race possess characteristics that are specific to that race, which distinguish it as inferior or superior to other races. This can lead individuals to be prejudiced towards someone for no reason other than their race. White supremacists believe white-skinned people are superior to other racial groups and aspire to see a society in which they are dominant; Black supremacy groups hold similar views with regard to their superiority.

Racist views held by nurses can impact on the quality of service received by the patient. McNaught (1985) reviewed accounts by Black and minority ethnic patients in hospital. He found:

- Minority ethnic patients were often left waiting unnecessarily and some staff made racists comments within earshot. Patients were sometimes addressed in a disrespectful manner.

- There were accounts of off-hand treatment and racist slurs by nurses. In mental health services the over-medication of patients was considered to be racially motivated.

The introduction of ADP should lead to an improvement in the unacceptable practices outlined above.

Exercise 16.4

Think about what measures you could take to learn about racism and how it may affect your work or practice. Do you question racist jokes and slurs when you hear them?

Ageism

When a person's age is used as an indicator of their competence or worth then *ageism* may be occurring. It can affect both young and old people. Think about the following:

Mrs Johnson, a previously active and independent woman was admitted 2 weeks ago after a fall. You overhear a nurse say:

> I do not know what that Mrs Johnson's family are thinking of trying to get the old dear back to her house aged 92? She will never manage. Best place for her is in residential care.

Or this to a woman aged 85 with Alzheimer's disease:

> Now then Queenie, my lovely, don't get all flustered, you sit down now and I will get you a drink. You just sit there dearie, be a good girl for me won't you.

Both examples above could be considered ageist. The first makes judgements about Mrs Johnson's ability based on her age. Her ability to go home would be determined by her physical and mental well-being and her own desire to live in a certain way.

Professor Queenie Gordon was treated like a child. An eminent academic she has written several books. The language used by the home manager in her exchange with Professor Gordon was demeaning.

Old age should not always be equated with frailty and vulnerability. *Being old does not cancel out what went before.*

Be alert to discrimination. If a gay, bisexual or lesbian patient is the subject of gossip, or given less good nursing *because of their sexual orientation*, then *homophobia* may be occurring. *Disablism can* occur when no allowances are made for the particular need of people with disability, when people behave differently towards them because of it.

16.4 Understanding emotional and sexual boundaries

Often people meet at work and go on to develop a personal relationship outside work. Consenting adults are free to make such decisions.

By contrast, sexual and emotional relationships between health workers (including students) and patients and clients are not permissible. Chapter 15 drew your attention to the statement in the Code (2008), which refers to this.

The responsibility for working within clear sexual and emotional boundaries rests with the professional, not with the patient/client. The Council for Health Care Regulatory Excellence (CRHE 2008:15) state that:

Breaches of sexual boundaries by health professionals are unacceptable, unprofessional and potentially unlawful.

The following are not acceptable behaviours if they occur between any professional, including students and patients/clients:

- Asking for or accepting a date.
- Sexual humour during consultation or examinations.
- Sexual or demeaning comments.
- Clinically irrelevant questions, e.g. about sexual orientation, their body or underwear.
- Requesting details of sexual orientation, history or preferences.
- Asking for, or accepting, an offer of sex.
- Watching a patient undress, *unless* a justified part of an examination.
- Taking or keeping photographs of the patient/client or their family that are not clinically necessary.
- Disclosing details of personal preferences, sexual problems, fantasies or other intimate details.
- Clinically unjustified physical examinations.

For further details see (Halter *et al.* 2007), available from: **www.chre.org.uk.**

Why are boundaries important?

Research shows (Halter *et al.* 2007) that significant and enduring harm can come to patients and clients as a result of sexualized behaviour by healthcare workers. Such behaviour can damage the patient's trust in the service and the public confidence in the professionalism of the staff. Additionally such behaviour can cloud professional judgement and influence decision-making.

Exercise 16.5 Discuss the situation below with some of your classmates and if necessary seek advice from your personal tutor.

You are working in an orthopaedic ward and have just accompanied your mentor as she gave some distressing news to a 22-year-old patient (the opposite sex to you). When the patient begins to cry you put your arm around them.

Is this touching acceptable? How may the patient feel when you touch them? Are certain touches more acceptable than others (e.g. a pat on the hand)? How would you know if the patient felt uncomfortable with your touch? What other method could be used to show concern and care? What should you do if a patient asks for a hug or a kiss? What should you do if the patient attempts to hug or kiss you?

There are no easy answers to these questions and each incident should be considered on its own merit. It is human nature to want to comfort someone in distress and between friends this is often done by touch. However, as a student nurse in a placement you must be cautious. In any interaction be aware of how it could be construed by the patient and of your intention. If you feel unsure, speak with your mentor or personal tutor.

Nurse teacher comment

66 It is *not* the aim of the pre-registration nursing programme to train out of students the human feelings of kindness, care and compassion so that sensitive incidents are managed in a cold, detached way. But neither must a nurse's own feelings impair their ability to perform the role. I think the balance is sensitive and considerate practice, which can empathize with the circumstances, at the same time as being effective and professional. 99

What if a patient or carer is attracted to you?

Dealing with such situations requires maturity and self-awareness. As a student, if you have any inclination that this may be occurring, then discuss it with your mentor or personal tutor. You must take the necessary action to avoid a breach of sexual boundaries. You should never interpret such behaviour as an opportunity to begin a sexual relationship.

What if you are attracted to patient or carer?

Talk with your mentor and ask for advice. A skilled mentor will be sensitive and ensure that another nurse takes over the care of this patient. Do not ignore the feelings and hope they will go away; they may not and the situation may develop. Acting on such feelings will have serious consequences for you and could lead to you being asked to leave the programme.

What should you do if you witness another student or health care professional breaching sexual boundaries?

The well-being of the patient is your primary concern. As soon as possible tell your mentor or the nurse in charge what you have seen. If the person concerned *is* your mentor, tell the nurse in charge or your personal tutor.

16.5 Barriers to good communication in practice

Good communication is an essential nursing skill but at times it is very difficult to achieve. Knowing some of the barriers to good communication can help and the next section highlights some of these. Remember to avoid the use of jargon. A patient may be perplexed to hear that you are looking for the landmarks for the dorsogluteal site, and content to know that you will give them an intramuscular injection in their bottom!

Speaking with a client can be impeded by television or other noise. Finding a quiet place (if you can) will help.

When communicating with people who have a limited understanding of English, avoid speaking too loudly; this does not aid understanding. Avoid slang, jargon and medical terms. Using non-verbal communication can help; gesture, point, use pictures, etc.

Be considerate when speaking with someone who is hard of hearing. They may lip read, so speak slowly and clearly. If you can, learn some basic skills in alternative communications, such as finger spelling or Makaton (for more details see: **www.makaton.org**).

The following tips may be helpful for your practice, and be particularly useful when working with vulnerable adults:

- Always start by assuming a person has the ability to understand what you are saying.
- Use a person's name to get their attention.
- Short, single sentences with one main idea are best. Don't give too much information at once.
- Avoid complex sentences that include negatives, abstract concepts, complex time dimensions, obscure expressions.
- Be respectful of age (only use the name preferred by the patient and no other).
- Be consistent in your vocabulary (lavatory, toilet, bathroom, ladies, gents). Use the language the person uses, if you know it.
- Communicate all the time! Understanding is enhanced through frequent exposure.
- Talk to the person, even if they cannot reply due to ill health or disability.
- Pace it right for the individual.
- Supplement spoken word with gestures, cues.
- Read body language, notice anxiety, distraction.
- Test for understanding, e.g. by asking the person to repeat back to you the advice you have given.

Communication is an essential nursing skill; practice makes perfect!

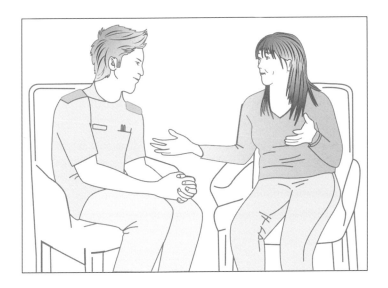

Figure 16.1 Talking to a client. Artist: Emma Heaton

16.6 Working with clients who lack mental capacity

Wherever you are in placement it is possible that some of the adult (16+) patients whom you nurse may lack mental capacity. This means they are unable to make a decision at the time it needs to be taken. It may be because they are ill, unconscious, affected by drugs or alcohol, have a learning disability or for any other reason (Mental Capacity Act 2005). A person is considered unable to make a decision if they cannot:

- Understand relevant information.
- Retain that information.
- Weigh up the information in reaching a decision.
- Communicate the decision.

Nurses must *always start by assuming a person has capacity* and, if in doubt, take all practical steps to support the person to make a decision. If after this a person is assessed as lacking capacity, all actions taken by others must be in the person's *best interests*. When a person lacks capacity and there is no family or friend to consult, an independent mental capacity advocate (IMCA) may be called to the ward to represent the person (DCA 2005). It is imperative that patients who lack capacity get the care they need; those who are unable to say they would like a drink must not go without. If you are concerned that patients you are nursing lack capacity, seek guidance from your mentor.

> **•••** **A word about** The Mental Capacity Act *deprivation of liberty safeguards* (DOLS)
>
> These safeguards provide legal protection for the most vulnerable people. They ensure a person receives the care and treatment that they need where, in their best interests, it is necessary to keep them safe. For more information see DOLS code of practice from: **www.publicguardian.gov.uk**.

16.7 **When a patient dies**

You do not need this book to tell you that such times can be difficult for all concerned. If you are working in a placement where you know it is possible that someone will die, then it is wise to tell your mentor if you have not experienced this situation before. Take time to reflect on the situation afterwards and talk through it with your mentor. Further reading about death and dying will also be helpful.

> *Student comment*
>
> 66 An elderly gentleman arrested on the ward and resuscitation was not successful. I was shocked that the body was left on the ward for the whole of the shift. His face was covered in muck and this was not cleaned before the family saw him. I felt even in death he was given no dignity. 99

As in the student comment above, you *must* seek support if you find any aspects of practice upsetting or difficult. But remember, you are in the placement to learn, and managing death is an important role of a nurse. For example, to understand how registered nurses support the families of patients who are dying and what activities must be performed once the person has died?

Being sensitive to their grief, *and only if your mentor agrees*, try to observe what is done both for the person that has died and for their relatives, family and friends. Note how it is considered important for relatives to see the deceased where they died. It helps them become closer to the event and be a part of it.

Mentor comment

❝ You may find seeing someone who has died quite difficult and need the support of your mentor. If this is the case, ask for the time you need and talk through your feelings. It may also help to write a reflection about the experience. ❞

What else will happen?

Traditionally, nurses will perform 'last offices', where the body is washed and wrapped, ready to be transported to the mortuary or funeral directors. This is a very important part of nursing practice. It is the final task that you can perform for a patient and should be done with great care and consideration.

Dying with dignity

Few people would wish to spend their last days in a hospital. Where this happens nurses have a duty to 'treat people as individuals and protect their dignity' and this includes at the point of death (NMC 2008: 2). Contrast the student experience below with the one above.

Student comment

❝ I had the privilege to meet a patient and her family just at the end of her life. All care was taken with providing the family a private place to go. The patient was in a six-bedded ward, which could have made things difficult; however, the staff provided the family members with pegs to put onto the curtains ... yes pegs ... I was very impressed with the ingenuity shown... they worked extremely well just holding the curtains closed where perhaps they would have gaped. ❞

Other difficult incidents

Various other difficulties can arise when patients or their families become very angry (or in rare cases, violent). In mental health settings, patients who are suicidal need vigilant observation. In a learning disability setting, witnessing a client having an epileptic seizure can be distressing. Seeing children with profound disabilities or those who are terminally ill can provoke understandable feelings of sadness. These are all circumstances that you may deal with in the future once you are a registered nurse. Take the time you need now, as a student, to think about these issues, observe how they are managed, so that when your time comes to take charge you will do so with confidence.

Summary

This chapter has raised your awareness to some of the challenging areas you may encounter and has challenged you to question yourself about whether you have the necessary value base for this work. Will you be alert to the needs of vulnerable people and treat all your patients equally and fairly leaving any personal feelings you may have at home? These questions are important as they say a lot about how you will deliver care to patient and clients, as well as something about your personal and professional development and your ethical practice. Progressing well in all these areas will be important for your success in your chosen field of practice, which the last chapter will now discuss.

■ Top tips

- Vulnerable people can sometimes react in ways that challenge nurses: it is not personal.
- Expect the course to challenge you from time to time.
- Be alert to the danger of behaviour that is out of bounds with clients and patients.
- Always be courteous, but do not say *too much* about yourself to patients and clients; if they ask, politely change the subject.
- Old, gay, opposite sex and disabled patients have the equal right to good quality care from nurses, and this includes you.
- Do not collude with any negative behaviour you may encounter.
- Respect the dignity of all patients.

■ Online resource centre

To get more advice on the challenges you might face, visit the website for the Council for Health Care Regulatory Excellence and read through the MCA code of practice. Links to where you can get this information can be found at: **www.oxfordtextbooks.co.uk/orc/hart**.

References

Council for Health Care Regulatory Excellence (2008: 15) *Learning about sexual boundaries between healthcare professionals and patients*. CHCRE, London.

Department for Constitutional Affairs (2005) Mental Capacity Act 2005 Code of Practice. The Stationery Office, Norwich, UK.

Halter M, Brown H and Stone J (2007) *Sexual boundary violations by health employees: an overview of the published empirical literature*. Council for Health Care Regulatory Excellence.

McNaught A (1985) *Race and health care in the United Kingdom*. Occasional Paper 2, Health Education Council, London.

Nursing and Midwifery Council (2008) the code standards of conduct, performance and ethics for nurses and midwires: **http://www.nmc_uk.org/aArticle.aspx?ArticleID=3056**.

Ministry of Justice (2008) *Deprivation of liberty safeguards: code of practice to supplement the main Mental Capacity Act 2005 Code of Practice*. The Stationery Office, Norwich, UK.

Mental Capacity Act (2005) **www.opsi.gov.uk/acts/acts2005/ukpga_20050009_en_1**.

Thompson N (2006) *Anti-discriminatory practice*, 4th edn. Palgrave Macmillan, Basingstoke.

Further reading

Holland K and Hogg C (2001) *Cultural awareness in nursing and health care: an introductory text*. Arnold, London.

17

Moving on!

Sue Hart

The aims of this chapter are:

➤ To assess your own progress so far

➤ To help you to know what will be expected in your chosen field of practice

➤ To introduce the concept of *transferability* of knowledge and skills

➤ To help keep you steady if things are going wrong

This last chapter will help you to prepare for the move into your field of practice. Starting the second year is different from starting the first. In a 3- (or more) year programme, the next stage will always be built on what has gone before. For example, in year two it will be assumed that you understand the topics you covered in year one. As a brand-new student, few assumptions were made about your knowledge and skills. Now, the sheet is no longer blank because, to be a second-year student, you must have:

• achieved all the entry to the branch outcomes in practice;

• achieved 120 credits at level 4 (Scotland level 7); and

• be progressing satisfactorily in your professional development.

17.1 Keeping on track: assessing your own progress so far

All students are different, and have their own personalities and abilities. Whilst respecting students as individuals, there are nevertheless certain characteristics that experienced nurse teachers can recognize in students who appear likely to succeed. Equally it is possible to recognize students who are struggling. Most universities require an end-of-year one report to be passed to the field of practice leaders. The following nurse teacher comments are brief extracts from such reports.

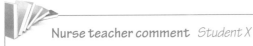

Nurse teacher comment *Student X*

66 Student: 'X' - Sept 2010 cohort Personal tutor: Sue Hart Date: 15/08/11

Theory: Achieved 48%, 53% and 61% for year 1 modules.

X was disappointed with her first mark and we discussed what she could do to improve her academic writing. I suggested she work through the university online study skills programme and that she reads more. She understands that in her first essay she relied too much on lecture material as evidence for her work. Her confidence has grown with the improving marks.

Practice: Reports from mentors have been positive. X is keen to learn whatever placement she is in and seeks opportunities to do new things. One mentor noted that she was 'open to learning and professional in her approach to patiens' and that she fitted well into the unit team.

Professional: X presents herself well. She is hard working and appears determined to do her best. She is a positive influence in the group both by contributing to discussions and listening to others. Although twice late for the 9.00am lecture in the same week (child care problems) she emailed an apology to the teacher and copied me as PT.

Sickness and absence: X has no recorded absences from class. She has had 7 consecutive days sickness (medical certificate provided).

Summary: X has made a steady start to the programme and if she continues to apply herself to her academic work she could do well in the second year, even though she knows the step up to level 5 studies may stretch her. Her professional development is good; she is very conscientious and responsible in all aspects of her work. 99

Nurse teacher comment *Student Y*

66 Student: 'Y' - Sept 2010 cohort Personal tutor: Debbie Roberts Date: 15/08/11

Theory: 'Y' has successfully completed 2 modules with marks of 42%, 46%. Has failed the exam for module 3 twice (18%, 32%) but has been given a third attempt. Re-sat on 29th July, result due next week. Heard today he did not attend the retrieval tutorial for the exam. Y was given (at his request) a 4-week extension for module 2 assignment (personal problems) and so submitted only two weeks before the first attempt at the exam. He insisted a 2-week extension would not be long enough – despite advice to the contrary.

Practice: Reports from Y's mentors are not encouraging. His mentor on an LD unit had to talk to him about his lateness and also for reading a newspaper when he » should have been observing a client. On placement 2 medical ward he needed reminding about his time-keeping and his appearance (muddy shoes). Link tutor held a three-way meeting with Y and the mentor to address this. His time-keeping improved on his 3rd placement, but there were problems with the overuse of his mobile 'phone.

Professional: Y is struggling on the programme. In discussion he does seem to understand where he makes mistakes, but does not sustain this in practice.

Y must reconsider his attitude and show commitment to the programme if he is going to succeed. He struggles academically and will need to apply himself more if he is to be successful in year 2. I will see him for a personal tutorial (assuming he passes the 3rd attempt and is not asked to leave for reasons of academic failure).

Sickness and absence: Y has 11 recorded absences from class. He has had 6 days sickness on 5 occasions (one episode of 2 days and 4 single days).

Summary: Y is not performing well at the moment and without more application to his work I fear he is unlikely to succeed. 〞

Exercise 17.1

First please re-read the above nurse teacher comments, underlining the strengths that X's personal tutor has reported and the concerns raised by Y's performance.

Now use the same headings to do a similar exercise yourself, *anticipating* what your personal tutor may be writing about you. Ask yourself honestly, are you succeeding? If not, talk to someone, *today*.

Nurse teacher comment

〝 Your teachers will consider you are succeeding if you have passed all the theory and practice assessments and show signs of developing in the profession. Note that success is different to 'high-flying'. Some students in your group may be getting top marks in everything they do (if you are one of them well done). If you are not, do not be disheartened or feel you are not achieving: if you have passed everything so far, you are. 〞

At this point hopefully you are on track with the course. If you are struggling, think about where you are failing; is it in theory, practice or with regards to your professional development?

17.2 **How will learning in year two be different?**

+ . . . .

Exercise 17.2

Please pause for a moment and recall the three essential skills sets that have featured in the book. How do you feel you have performed in each so far?

. . . .

Naturally, what is *expected* of a second-year student is more advanced than what is expected of a first year, and how you will *feel* as a second-year student will differ because of the experience you have now had. By the end of year one, you should recognize how *the three essential skills sets merge*.

Remember, at any one time a registered nurse is:

- drawing on her knowledge and thinking about what she is doing (theory and reflection);
- using nursing skills and delivering nursing care;
- acting within the bounds of her professional role and observing the NMC Code.

So, in reality it is clear that, unlike the image in Chapter 1, the three essential skills sets should be presented like that seen in Figure 17.1.

If you are to perform well in the second year you must be able to *transfer* your learning so far and apply it to new situations.

Transferability of knowledge

Transferability refers to how you are expected to *carry with you, apply, build on and develop* the learning you have had so far on the programme, to each new area in which you are placed and to the assignments and other written work you are required to do.

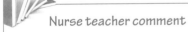

Nurse teacher comment

" Remember, your field-of-practice leaders and mentors don't know you well yet but they know what they *expect* of you.... It will help your success to perform at the level they expect. "

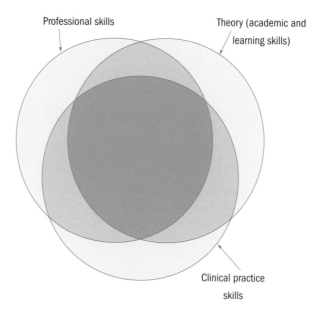

Figure 17.1 Diagram of three skills sets overlapping

17.3 Advancing your learning and academic skills

In Chapter 5 we used Bloom's theory of learning to show how students develop through the programme. In the second year and beyond, you will be expected to develop and perform at the higher levels illustrated in italics in Table 17.1. Think of yourself as working towards this level of performance.

Assignments

Please look at the level 5 (level 8 Scotland) grading criteria at your university and compare with that for the first year. Note how what is expected of your work will change. These changes will be reflected in your assignment guidelines. See this example of a level-5 child branch module assessment question.

> An essay discussing a child nursing intervention, *exploring and critiquing the evidence-base* for the intervention. The essay should include the *quality of the evidence, leadership and management* issues, e.g. change-management, legal and ethical issues, and personal and professional development. (3000 words)

Note the key words: critiquing (a detailed analysis and assessment); quality (the standard of something as measured against other things of a similar kind). These words are not the same as 'outline' and 'describe'!

Domain	Concerned with:	Moving from the simple to the more complex					
Cognitive	Knowledge	Recall data	Understand	*Apply*	*Analyse*	*Synthesis*	*Evaluation*
Psychomotor	Skills	Copy	Follow instructions	*Develop percision*	*Combine related skills*	*Become expert*	
Affective	Attitude	Awareness	React	*Value*	*Organize*	*Adopt behaviour*	

Table 17.1 Anticipated student nurse journey of development from the second year to the end of the programme (adapted from the work of Bloom 1956).

Evidenced-based practice (EBP)

As you know, this means that practice is based on knowledge, nursing research and professional standards of care. A nurse should always understand why they are delivering each nursing care intervention, the rationale for their action and the consequences of acting differently, or failing to act. In the second year and beyond, it is essential that you show in your written work (as well as in practise) that you understand this important principle. See Holland and Rees (2010) for a more in-depth understanding of EBP.

Marking

By now it will be expected that you have dealt with any difficulties you may have had with writing, grammar, punctuation and referencing. In the early days, your teachers may have helped you by *correcting* your errors. Do not automatically expect this to happen later.

Important note

If, after completing some of the first-year assignments, you feel you may have a specific learning need (e.g. dyslexia), talk to your personal tutor about this. Some students are not assessed until well into the course.

New class

In year two you will be taught mostly by lecturers from your own field of practice background and references to practice will be branch specific. Prepare to engage in your learning with discussions and more group work. The more you read, the more you will get from your learning. Interact with the lecturers; like mentors they expect to be questioned by students. *Year two students are expected to be active learners, not passive recipients of information.*

17.4 Showing your professional development in clinical practice placements

Your first day in practice as a second-year student will feel different to that in your first year. What will have felt new and strange, e.g. people calling you 'student nurse', is now familiar. You will no longer be one of the most junior students. Your mentor will expect that you can, under supervision, perform some basic nursing care activities with confidence (although do not be offended if a new mentor wants to see you perform a skill before they let you do it at arm's length). Also, if a first-year student is on your placement that, under the supervision of your mentor, you guide them in some basic activities and help them to settle. See this as part of your development.

Exercise 17.3

Revisit Chapter 15 now if you are unsure why you should see the last point as part of your development. The answer is there.

In the second-year placements, it would be usual for your mentor to be on the same part of the register as that you are studying towards. As before, they will help facilitate your learning and ensure you have learning experiences to meet your assessment criteria. They will not expect to have to guide you by the hand to achieve your learning outcomes, but to direct and support you to do so. Through direct observation of you in the placement, they will assess your competence and ensure that you practice safely and effectively.

Paperwork

In your first placements allowances would have been made for some initial confusion; the paperwork can be complex. Now, you should be familiar with what is expected of you to complete your assessment of practice.

Professional behaviour

Chapters 14 and 15 explained in detail the standard of professionalism required of registered nurses. Not performing well in the basics of professional behaviour is more serious for a second-year student. It should by now be second nature to you to be reliable, trustworthy, correctly dressed and punctual. Your attention should be moving towards developing your *ethical practice*, e.g. showing that you understand *why* there is a need to treat patients respectfully, rather than just knowing you should.

It will help your success to show that you understand and accept the additional level of responsibility that comes with being a second-year student, especially in taking responsibility for working well with your mentor, engaging in the programme and seeking out learning opportunities for yourself.

Recording your own progress

Your nurse teachers will have advised you what evidence you will need for your sign-off mentor at the end of the programme (as explained in Chapter 13). It is essential you do this carefully, as failure to produce the evidence may delay your completion of the programme.

> **! Fact box**
>
> From the beginning of the second year you will be working towards the NMC (2004) standards of proficiency for *entry to the register*.

Reflective diary/journal

As suggested in Chapter 12, there is much to gain from keeping such a diary, whether it is a requirement for your course or not. As you progress through the course, looking back to see how you felt, thought, reacted to a situation earlier can help you recognize your development (and often raise a smile).

Personal development planning (PDP)

Personal development planning refers to a process designed to support you to manage your studies, improve your career prospects and support your professional development. Most universities have such a process for all students, not only nursing students. It is increasingly recognized that understanding *how* you are learning, as well as *what* you are learning, has a positive impact on success. PDP can help you to:

- do well in your studies by helping you to think about what you want to achieve and what you need to get there;
- plan your development by helping you to identify your skills and abilities;
- identify how the skills developed can be transferred to employment situations;
- plan your career by helping you to think about your options;
- help you build up a record of experiences and achievements;
- prepare you for life beyond university.

Broadly, the activity involves the setting of long- and short-term goals with regular self-assessment and review of progress. Students are encouraged to set goals using

SMART language. This acronym stands for Specific, Measurable, Achievable, Realistic and Timed.

17.5 Why students leave pre-registration nursing courses (and how not to become a statistic)

The Department of Health published a report in September 2006 'Managing attrition rates for student nurses and midwives'. It is available to read electronically (see below). Statistically, male students and younger students are more likely to leave, as well as older students who have not studied for some time. Part-timers leave more frequently than full-timers. If you fit into one or more of these categories, ensure you get the help you need for your particular circumstances. The transition to university life can be hard when you are young (maybe away from home for the first time and especially if you are finding the course challenging).

- There is no shame in saying you are finding it hard. The university does not want you to leave and often will be able to direct you to support that you did not know could be available.

The health service needs nurses who reflect the cultural backgrounds of the patients and clients who receive services and universities welcome eligible students who are likely to be successful on the programme, irrespective of their origins. Nevertheless, some students can find the course and the clinical nursing practise a challenge.

- Make sure you tell your personal tutor if there are culturally sensitive reasons that may affect your practise. It is much better to be open about issues before you are in placement and work to find a solution.

The report also found that poor attendance on the programme was problematic and can lead to academic failure.

Nurse teacher comment

❝ I remember a student who used to get good marks. She came unstuck though when she failed to attend a series of lectures and missed the module 'surgery', where I went through what was expected in the assignment. Her essay made the fundamental mistake that I warned the students not to make. She had to resubmit. It brought her down to earth with a bang. ❞

Hopefully, you will experience being allocated to a good team, with an excellent mentor. It is also possible that you may be placed in an area that you perceive as less dynamic. As you know from the media, the quality of care in the health service can vary. Many staff work in very difficult circumstances and under huge pressure.

- It helps to remember that, if you are not enjoying a placement as much as you have others, it will only be for a limited time. It is unlikely that you will enjoy every place-ment as much as your favourites; it is fine to have a preference. For the purpose of the programme you *must* have the variety of experience; so accept, engage, learn, move on. Remember also, that although learning from positive role models is good, learning does occur in all settings.

You should have been told at interview that not all placements will necessarily be on your doorstep and Chapter 7 of this book explained why. If travelling is getting you down what can you do?

- If this is the case, point out to your personal tutor that you have had several place-ments with a lot of travelling. Ask if it is possible to negotiate doing more hours in practice for fewer days per week to make the most of the journey. Again, remember it is not forever. *Don't let a few difficult journeys get in the way of your ambition to be a nurse.* Also do not think if you did the course elsewhere it would solve the problem as *all courses* require some travelling.

If you have specific difficulties (e.g. financial difficulties, emotional problems or family pres-sures) you are advised to speak to your personal tutor.

- If you have money difficulties revisit the advice in Chapter 3. Your personal tutor may be able to offer support or recommend a counsellor to help you through any other difficulties. Many students have enormous challenges when on the course and help is at hand. Do not assume your problem is so big you have no alterative but to leave *before* discussing your situation with someone.

If you become pregnant when you are on the course, for your own well-being and that of your unborn child you *must* tell your personal tutor or the course leader at the earliest pos-sible opportunity. You have the right to ask this individual that your privacy is respected.

- You need to be aware that in clinical practice there are risks and hazards, which must be assessed if you are pregnant, e.g. the risk of musculoskeletal injuries as a result of lifting is higher during pregnancy. Also, fatigue can result from prolonged physical activity. You will be supported to stay on the programme as long as it is safe for you to do so. If you can time your departure for maternity leave with the ending of a module, this will make your return easier.

The Department of Health report (2006) found some students left their nursing programme because they were unhappy with the organization and management at the university they attended.

- If you are in such a situation, there is a lot you can do. Programme leaders *do not know what it feels like to be a student on their course*, but you can be 100% confident that, if they are getting something wrong, they will want to know in order that they can put it right. So talk to them. *Remember they want the same result as you: your success.* Take your concerns to your personal tutor, student representative (as mentioned in Chapter 2) or put them face-to-face or in writing to the programme lead.

If you are ill you must ensure you provide the university with certificates for your time away.

- If your ill health is prolonged, then stepping off the course and returning to complete is possible (see Chapter 2).

Lastly, if academic failure is your problem, please re-read the relevant section in Chapters 5 or 6.

Nurse teacher comment

❝ If you wish (or have to) leave before you complete the course, please leave well! On no account just disappear. You will want a reference in the future and a transcript of the credits (CAT points) you have earned. Also, be aware that if you receive bursary payments after you have left, you will normally be expected to repay them. Attend the exit interview and return all university property, locker keys, library books and library cards, etc. and your name badge. You will be told if you have to return any uniforms. If you are choosing to leave, time your departure so it works to your favour, e.g. if your university awards a certificate at the end of the first year to students who have completed all the CFP successfully but then leave, you may get a higher education certificate on your CV and something to show for your study. That has got to be better than leaving with nothing. ❞

Summary

Having read this book you are now well-positioned to know exactly what is required of you to achieve on the pre-registration nursing course through the first year and into the second. Your success from here is down to you. Take all the learning with you and most of all *enjoy the rest of the course.*

Student comment

❝ Above all have a good time. The student nurse time is one of the best parts of your nursing life; you have the privilege of being supernumerary, so use it to your advantage. The friends that you make now will probably be with you for a long time. Good luck. ❞

▪ Top tips

- Time-management; know your deadlines and keep to them.
- Attend lectures. Listen and take good notes.
- Read around the subjects you are studying; this is *essential* when writing assignments.
- Aim to pass all your assessments at the first attempt. This avoids the need to re-sit, using time you need to complete your next assessment.
- Keep your personal tutor informed of any circumstances that may be distracting you from the course.
- Make friends with 'good' students who are working hard and determined to succeed. Associate yourself with success.
- Give time-wasters and people who miss (or worse still *disrupt* lectures) a wide berth.
- Be reliable and flexible in practice and care for children, patients and clients as you would wish someone you cared about to be nursed.
- Make an effort to communicate well with your mentor.
- Learn from constructive criticism and feedback. Learn not to take it to heart. Listen, learn and move on. Do not bear grudges.
- Listen to guidance from your teachers and mentors, be respectful of their experience.
- Enjoy the course; that way you will learn well and succeed.

▪ Online resource centre

Get a good idea of how you are doing by looking at the level-2 grading criteria at: **www.oxfordtextbooks.co.uk/orc/hart/**. If there are areas you feel could be improved, go back through the sections in this book that will help you do so.

■ References

Bloom BS (1956) *Taxonomy of educational objectives*. Allyn and Bacon, Boston, MA. Copyright © 1984 by Pearson Education.

Department of Health (2006) *Managing attrition rates for student nurses and midwives: a guide to good practice for strategic health authorities and higher education institutions*. (Gateway reference 7609). Crown Copyright: **http://www.dh.gov.uk/prod_consum_dh/groups/dh_digitalassets/ @dh/@en/documents/digitalasset/dh_073226.pdf**

Holland K and Rees C (2010) in Nursing: Evidence-based practical learning skills. Oxford University Press, Oxford.

Nursing and Midwifery Council (2004) *Standards of proficiency for pre-registration nursing education*. Standards 02 04. NMC, London.

Nursing and Midwifery Council (2008) *The code: standards of conduct, performance and ethics for nurses and midwives*. NMC, London.

■ Further reading

Kubler-Ross E (1969) *On death and dying*. Macmillan, New York.
A classic text on the subject.

■ Websites

An excellent tutorial on critical thinking and critical reading: **http://unilearning.uow.edu.au/ critical/**

A step-by-step discussion of how to integrate critical analysis within your essays: **http://www. palgrave.com/skills4study/pdfs/critical%20analysis%20.pdf#search=%22critical% 20analysis%20palgrave%22**

Edwards SL (1998) Critical thinking and analysis: a model for written assignments. *British Journal of Nursing* **7**(3): 159–166. Available from: **http://www.internurse.com/cgi-bin/go.pl/library/ article.cgi?uid=5768&article=BJN_7_3_159_166**

Department of Health 2006 Guide to Managing attrition rates for student nurses and midwives: **http://www.dh.gov.uk/en/Publicationsandstatistics/Publications/PublicationsPolicyAnd Guidance/DH_073230**

Glossary

A

Affective domain Affective refers to attitudes and feelings. The affective domain is one part of Bloom's taxonomy.

B

Best interests Any decisions made, or anything done for a person who lacks capacity must be in the person's best interests.

Branch/field of practice Practice may be within one of four areas of nursing: adult, child, learning disabilities or mental health. The term field of practice is replacing the term branch to refer to these.

C

Capacity The ability to make a decision about a particular matter at the time the decision needs to be made.

Cognitive domain Cognitive relates to cognition, the mental process of acquiring knowledge and understanding. The cognitive domain is one part of Bloom's taxonomy.

Cohort Another name for a 'group' or 'set' or 'class' or 'intake' of student nurses. All these terms are in use.

Colonoscopy A test enabling a doctor to look directly at the lining of the large bowel.

Common Foundation Programme (CFP) The current NMC term for the first year of the nursing programme. From September 2011 the term is to be dropped and replaced with *first year*.

Competence An ability to do something well. In nursing this refers to the skills and abilities to practise safely and effectively.

Cystic fibrosis A life-threatening inherited disease that affects the internal organs by clogging them with thick, sticky mucous (see more at: cftrust.org.uk)

E

Enquiry-based learning (EBL)/problem-based learning (PBL) These are student-led learning strategies commonly used on nursing programmes. A group of students are given a topic and then must research answers to questions raised.

Epilepsy A neurological disorder marked by abnormal activity in the brain often resulting in seizures (fits) of various types.

European Directive (ED) A legislative act of the European Union. There are EDs concerning adult nursing.

Evidence-based practice Where nursing interventions are based on knowledge and research. This keeps practice up-to-date.

G

Guidelines A generic (catch all) term used in this book for information given to you by your university. They may be guidelines for writing assignments, or a list of what you can and cannot do in practice. You are advised always to read any guidelines given and file them for future reference.

H

Health care assistant (HCA) Works under the supervision of a registered nurse team leader and assists in the delivery of health care and clinical tasks. Activities vary according to the environment and may include, supporting people to eat and drink, washing and dressing. When trained, HCAs can also perform additional tasks such as blood pressure monitoring and urinalysis.

Life-long learning Registered nurses have a professional duty to keep up-to-date. This is known as continuing professional development (CPD). This life-long learning can be through post-registration courses, as well as self-directed. The academic and study skills you learn during the pre-registration programme will prepare you for this.

M

Mainstream services In relation to people with learning disability this means services everyone uses (e.g. local swimming pool), rather than facilities particularly designed for people with disabilities, which are known as *specialist* services. Mainstream is good; it means people with learning disability are out in the community and not segregated.

Makaton A language programme using signs and symbols in use widely by people with learning disability and their carers.

Marking/moderation Normally course work is marked by one teacher, then passed to another teacher for a second mark, and then to a team of teachers who moderate the whole batch of marking. A sample of scripts will be third marked as well. This is done to ensure fairness.

Mentor A person, most often a registered nurse, who supervises and assesses students in practice.

Multi-disciplinary team Where several professionals from different disciplines work together. Sometimes known as *multi-agency* (i.e. professionals from different agencies, e.g health, social care, housing).

N

Nursing and Midwifery Council (NMC) The NMC is the regulatory body for nursing and midwifery. (See more about the role of the NMC in Chapter 14.)

National vocational qualifications (NVQs) NVQs are work-related, competence-based qualifications.

P

Plagiarism Taking someone else's work or ideas and passing them off as your own.

Portfolio These are documents you create that contain the evidence you have met the learning required of you in practice. (See Chapter 13 for more about portfolios.)

Project 2000 The name of first pre-registration nursing programme to lead to an academic award of Diploma in Higher Education, which moved pre-registration nursing education from the NHS into the higher education sector. These programmes were introduced from 1989.

Psychomotor skills Nurses use psycho-motor skills when carrying out certain nursing practise skills with patients, such as giving an injection. (Psycho) conscious mental activity in movement or action (motor).

R

Reflection This is a developmental activity. A tool for thinking about what you do and learning from it. Chapter 12 will develop your understanding of reflective practice.

S

Special-care baby units (SCBU) A baby may be transferred here for specialist care, e.g. after a difficult delivery, or if they are born small, or following complex surgery.

Spider diagram or map So named, because it resembles a spider's web. Creating such diagrams allows for more flexibility than linear note-taking. The 'body' of the spider represents the main topic, with the 'legs' representing related themes or concepts. Creating such diagrams can help bring focus to a topic, can aid a review of the topic and enable a student to monitor their growing comprehension. It can also help highlight areas requiring more work, by identifying areas where the web is hard to complete.

Sponsored/commissioned students These are usually mature students who are employed by an NHS Trust, e.g. as a healthcare assistant, and who have now been sponsored to undertake the pre-registration nursing course.

Step off Where a student leaves the programme for a period of time (e.g. due to illness) and returns to join a later group.

University The NMC often refer to universities as HEIs. This means Higher Education Institutes.

Index